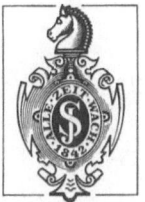

Wolfgang P. E. Raab

The Treatment of Mycosis with Imidazole Derivatives

Foreword by A. M. Kligman

Translated by T. C. Telger

With 41 Figures and 19 Tables

Springer-Verlag
Berlin Heidelberg New York 1980

Univ. Professor Dr. WOLFGANG P. E. RAAB
3, Walfischgasse, A-1010 Vienna

Translator: TERRY C. TELGER
3054 Vaughn Avenue, Marina, CA 93933, USA

Title of the original German edition 1978:
Mykosebehandlung mit Imidazolderivaten (Kliniktaschenbücher)

ISBN-13 : 978-3-540-09800-3   e-ISBN-13 : 978-3-642-67508-9
DOI: 10.1007/978-3-642-67508-9

Library of Congress Cataloging in Publication Data: Raab, Wolfgang. The treatment of mycosis with imidazole derivatives.   Translation of Mykosebehandlung mit Imidazolderivaten. Includes bibliographical references and index.   1. Mycoses-Chemotherapy. 2. Imidazole-Therapeutic use. 3. Antifungal agents. I. Title. RC117.R313   619.9'69'061   79-24361

Foreword

This is an "old-fashioned" book in the best sense of the term: It is written by *one* man, and it is scholarly, complete, thorough, and thoughtful. It is, in fact, a magnum opus wherein every aspect is not only touched, but handled to perfection. This is a treatise that deserves careful reading by that increasing cadre of medical specialists who understand the many ways in which mycoses threaten human health and happiness, viz, the veterinarian, pharmaceutical chemist, general practitioner, pharmacologist, and entire consortium of researchers who study the biology, epidemiology, pathogenesis, and treatment of fungus infections. Mycoses encompass a vast spectrum of diseases from trivial superficial skin infections (tinea versicolor), troublesome ringworm infections (the tineas of skin, hair, and nails), yeast infections (candidosis), the systemic mycosis (cryptococcosis, histoplasmosis), and even the deep-seated infections due to molds and saprophytic fungi (aspergillosis).

It is precisely because of the great variety of causative organisms that the imidazoles deserve a special treatise. They provide the first class of drugs with therapeutic activity against *all* the important fungi which infect humans and animals. Accordingly, their medical significance is great and the possibilities endless. Morever, the imidazoles are the first effective drugs whose antimicrobial activities extend beyond the usual designation of "broad-spectrum." Broad-spectrum antibiotics, for example, are either antifungal or antibacterial, not both as the imidazoles are. To be sure, there have been other chemotherapeutic compounds which inhibit bacteria and fungi. But these have been either toxic (phenol) or only marginally effective. For example, the quinolines (clioquinol, etc.) have broad-spectrum activity, and their topical use has been extensive for decades. However, their in vivo performance is unimpressive though useful while there was nothing better. In superficial ringworm and yeast infections, they generally moderate rather than cure. Raab, in his devotion to fairness, overrates the efficacy of the 8-hydroxyquinolines. Again, the dispassionate Raab, dealing with another broad-spectrum drug, haloprogin, defers an evaluation of efficacy, because clinical testing is still going on and the final place of the agent is uncertain. The fact is, however, that haloprogin is appreciably less effective than the imidazoles in the more stubborn ringworm infections. The marketplace in the United States has rendered this judgment unequivocally. Miconazole and clotrimazole formulations far outsell haloprogin.

The imidazoles are to the therapy of fungus infections what the corticosteroids were to the treatment of inflammatory dermatoses. They are revolutionary, novel, and have immense potential for further improvement by molecular manipulation. This class of compounds deserves emphasis, for therapeutic applications are certainly not limited to fungus infections. We must remember that certain imidazoles have been known for sometime to be effective antitrichomonads (metronidazole) and antihelmintics (thiabendazole). Standing apart from all the other anti-infective imidazoles is levamisole which has the remarkable property of enhancing immunologic responsiveness, especially of the cell-mediated variety.

New antifungal imidazoles are literally gushing out of the wells of pharmaceutical research. We scarcely grew acquainted with clotrimazole (the oldest) and miconazole, when new improved models came forth, e.g., isoconazole and econazole. And now etoconazole is being intensively studied for oral use. Others with special features are on the way.

It is in topical therapy that the benefits of the imidazoles have been very impressive indeed. The raison d'être for launching a drug into the channels of commerce is either greater efficacy or fewer hazards, that is, greater safety. The imidazoles satisfy both these requirements. They have only a slight potential for irritation and contact sensitization; besides, they are colorless and odorless. Systemic toxicity is likewise very low; hence, there is little danger of adverse effects, even with widespread application.

Does it matter that the imidazoles inhibit gram-positive bacteria? The answer is emphatically yes! Without this antimicrobial activity, the imidazoles would be decidedly less impressive topically, perhaps comparable to tolnaftate, a valuable agent in simple uncomplicated ringworm of the trunk. It must be remembered that fungus infections thrive in the wet, "tropical" regions of the body, notably between the toes and in the groin and perineum. Moisture and warmth also favor the luxuriant growth of bacteria, which may reach very high densities in these areas. These bacteria are, for the most part, ones which normally reside on the skin, mainly gram-positive cocci and diphtheroids. However, virulent streptococci and staphylococci can incite nasty secondary infections in hot climates where personal hygiene is difficult to maintain. In any event, the overgrowth of gram positives contributes significantly to the symptomatology – the itching, maceration, exudation, tenderness, and odor. Thus, antibacterial activity is a real asset.

Raab deals decisively with a controversial aspect of topical antimicrobial therapy, namely, combination with anti-inflammatory corticosteroids. Some academic purists condemn combinations, arguing that their use encourages "shot-gun" therapy and discourages accurate diagnosis. These debates delight the scholars but have little impact on front-line clinicians who must treat diseases without the backup laboratory. Besides, the patient cannot wait for the laboratory results. The fact is that physicians in general have very little training in dermatology and cannot be expected to appreciate the morphological fine points which enable the expert – but only sometimes – to tell when a ringworm infection is secondarily infected and when the diagnosis is moniliasis, not an unrelated rash. It is true enough that the various ringworm lesions will respond to a formulation containing a single imidazole such as econazole; still, the signs and symptoms will generally subside more swiftly when a corticosteroid is also present. Rapid relief is important to patients. Moreover, physicians deserve as much coverage as they can get. For short-term use, the worry about the adverse effects of corticosteroids is unjustified. Also, a variety of intertriginous lesions can resemble ringworm and moniliasis, e. g., seborrheic dermatitis. A mistaken diagnosis has little consequence. The corticosteroid will suppress the dermatitis. Raab shows clearly that corticosteroids and the imidazoles are compatible with each other.

A thorough account is given of the mode of action; killing is achieved by a disturbance of membrane permeability, upsetting transport of nutrients in and out of the cell. These alterations of the cell membranes and intra-cellular organelles are beautifully illustrated by marvelously informative scanning electron micrographs. Looking at these one can feel the distress of the fungi as they undergo anatomic disintegration.

Raab leaves nothing uncovered. The chemistry, toxicology, and pharmacology of the imidazoles are treated extensively. The clinician will find that this is also a textbook of medical mycology in which the diagnosis and treatment of fungus infections of all varieties are neatly and clearly presented.

As if the imidazoles were not meritorious enough, they have a further virtue in that, unlike antibiotics, there is little likelihood that the fungi will become resistant, requiring substitution of alternate drugs, an endless process of struggle.

Raab makes us aware that the drama of development of the imidazoles is still unfolding – that improved chemical species are ready for almost immediate use. Especially exciting in this regard is the long-awaited, safe, and effective treatment for health-destroying and occasionally fatal systemic infections. With amphotericin, for example, it is sometimes preferable to endure the disease rather than fight the dreadful toxic effects of the drug. Happily, the imidazoles can be given orally, intravenously, and intramuscularly and are usually well tolerated.

Because of their safety, efficacy and versatility, we can expect the pace of development to be swift. Raab's treatise is a great contribution to the library of medical mycology. This English edition is certain to be as well received as the earlier German one. Indeed, the subject is so important that we can expect Raab to prepare a revised, updated edition in less than five years!

ALBERT M. KLIGMAN

Preface to the English Edition

Imidazole derivatives receive increasing attention the world over as among them the most active broad-spectrum antifungal substances are found. In topical and systemic antifungal therapy, more and more use will be made of the imidazole derivatives. In the United States, sofar, only clotrimazole and miconazole are available for topical antifungal treatment. But that will change soon. Therefore, it seems appropriate to compile the information on antifungal imidazoles for English speaking readers. The German version which appeared in 1978 has been completely revised and the latest data from experimental investigations and clinical trials have been included in order to bring the information up to date, a most important point in such a quickly changing field as antifungal chemotherapy.

As the author, I am deeply indebted to Professor Albert Kligman, University of Pennsylvania in Philadelphia, for his continuing interest and help in the preparation of this book.

Vienna, January 1980   WOLFGANG P. E. RAAB

Preface to the German Edition

With the rise of microbial infections, especially those caused by various species of fungi, antimicrobial therapy is becoming increasingly important in all branches of medicine. Owing to its special pharmacologic properties and broad antimicrobial spectrum, one group of substances stands out from the rest: the imidazole derivatives, which include clotrimazole, miconazole and its stereoisomer isoconazole, as well as econazole and ketoconazole. These compounds are active not only against all types of fungi pathogenic to man, but also against gram-positive bacteria. For this reason they are also called *broad-spectrum antimicrobials.*

From the standpoint of the clinical pharmacologist, the use of imidazole derivatives for the treatment of mycoses of the skin and mucous membranes is highly welcome. The compounds indicated are well tolerated, and the risk of sensitization is extremely low. In only one case has the development of a clinically relevant resistance been observed. Imidazole derivatives can be incorporated into numerous vehicles, providing the therapist with lesion- and localization-specific modes of topical administration appropriate for all skin and mucous membrane changes.

The experimental testing and clinical investigation of clotrimazole and miconazole were followed by the latest introduction in the area of antimicrobial imidazole derivatives: econazole and ketoconazole. Practical experience with econazole in the *topical treatment* of mycosis has justified the optimism raised by the results of pharmacologic studies. Ketoconazole seems most promising for *systemic (oral) administration.*

Important new discoveries have been made in the area of skin-surface biology in recent years. The changes that occur in skin-surface microorganisms during various diseases and under the influence of various therapies have been the object of extensive research. From the results of such research, new principles have emerged for the treatment of chronic inflammatory skin lesions.

The worldwide increase in microbial infections of body surfaces, the changing concept of the importance of antimicrobial agents with regard to chronic inflammatory skin changes, and the improved therapeutic prospects created by a new class of substances suggest that new guidelines may be needed for the local treatment of microbial infections and secondary invasions ("colonizations").

XI

The purpose of this clinical handbook is to present a thorough discussion of the topical treatment of mycotic infections with imidazole derivatives, and of the theoretical and pharmacologic bases for the introduction of new therapeutic agents. The practicing physician and the medical researcher are given much-needed basic information on antimycotics and antimicrobials in general, based primarily on the drug econazole. The requirements of the clinical pharmacologist are given particular consideration. An attempt is also made to answer the controversial question of whether or not antimicrobial agents should be combined with glucocorticoids in topical therapy.

In its discussion of the latest antimicrobial drugs, this book seeks to summarize the principles which underlie the development of new topical antimicrobial agents. The practicing physician, in turn, must be shown what therapeutic results he may expect with such substances under optimal conditions. He is advised to determine for himself the results that can be achieved by the use of "optimal" agents in the treatment of mycotic infections. The introduction of imidazole derivatives has substantially broadened and enhanced the possibilities of local antimicrobial and especially antimycotic therapy. The reasons for this are set forth in this monograph. It is hoped that this book, like its predecessors, will serve to deepen the knowledge and understanding of the clinical application of newly developed drugs.

I am indebted to the following colleagues for supplying illustrations to the text: Dr. S. Ånséhn of Linköping (Fig. 7), Dr. M. Dorn of Munich (Fig. 31), Dr. D. Grigoriu of Lausanne (Figs. 30, 32b–d, 37a), Dr. H. J. Preusser of Darmstadt (Figs. 6, 14–19), Dr. H. Rieth of Hamburg (Figs. 39, 40), and Dr. B. Winblad of Umea (Fig. 7).

Vienna, June 1978   WOLFGANG P. E. RAAB

XII

Contents

1 Introduction

1.1 Antimicrobial Therapy

Every age has its own medicine and its own particular methods of treatment. The rise of chemistry which began in this century and has intensified in recent decades has led to profound changes in medical therapeutics. The development of ever newer drugs and modes of administration has brought continuous improvements. This applies to local therapy as well, for which a number of highly effective and convenient-to-use drugs are now available in vehicles appropriate for specific lesions. The number of drugs is already so large that it can scarcely be conceived. Often several drugs, usually supplied in various preparations, are offered for the same indications.

As the use of antibiotics and antimicrobials has increased, so has the frequency of adverse (unintended) effects in both local and systemic therapy. The adverse effects of drugs may be either *direct* or *indirect* (survey in [234, 247, 248]). The broad spectrum of the sometimes life-threatening *direct* adverse effects of drugs has become known only during the last two decades. In systemic therapy, the selection of the drug to be administered is now based not only on its efficacy, but also on the absence of adverse effects. This is particularly evident in the case of antibiotics. Even the local application of such agents is leading increasingly to problems associated with direct adverse effects. The main problem is the high incidence of *sensitization* that occurs during local treatment. If sensitization of the immediate type occurs during local treatment, the systemic administration of the same or a chemically similar drug later on may trigger a severe general reaction. For this reason many countries now prohibit locally applied antibiotics from being given systemically, and vice versa. Fortunately, the local application of drugs usually causes only a delayed sensitization; repeated application of the same drug leads only to an eczematous contact reaction (or exanthema). While such reactions significantly impair the state of the skin, they are seldom dangerous. Nevertheless, both the delayed and immediate reactions have tended to discourage the use of antibiotics in local therapy, with very few exceptions (e. g., erythromycin).

By comparison, *indirect* adverse drug reactions are more common during the local application of antimicrobials. Many antimicrobials, especially those with a narrow spectrum, lead to a *disturbance of the microbial balance,* which

1

promotes infection by pathogenic organisms that are not susceptible to the drug administered (see Sects. 9 and 10). A further problem is *resistance,* which pertains in particular to local therapy involving the exposure of microbes to insufficient concentrations of antimicrobial drugs. Comparative studies of the changes in the resistance behavior of skin-surface microorganisms, notably staphylococci [17, 124, 161, 196], indicate that the local application of antibiotics is becoming increasingly less effective. The therapist is faced with two facts: On the one hand, microbial infections are on the rise in all branches of medicine (see Sect. 9), and the need for safe, reliably effective antimicrobials (and antimycotics) is increasing; on the other hand, the efficacy of various drugs is reduced by pathogen resistance, and their applicability is limited by sensitization. As a result, ever newer antimicrobial agents are required in the interests of *safe* and *effective* treatment.

However, in order to break the vicious circle (new drug → sensitization and development of resistance → need for another new drug), increasing attention is being focused on the requirements of the clinical pharmocologist. New antimicrobials (and antimycotics) for local therapy should not only be highly effective and induce minimal resistance, but should also be nonsensitizing or at least have a sensitization index which is extremely low. According to previous observations, the family of antimicrobially active imidazole derivatives appears to satisfy these stringent requirements to a large degree (see Sect. 8) and has therefore led to a significant overall improvement in the topical treatment of the skin and mucous membranes for microbial (mycotic) infections.

1.2 Microbial Diseases of the Skin and Mucous Membranes

The presence of large numbers of microbes can regularly be detected on the human skin under normal conditions. This flora consists for the most part of staphylococci and other gram-positive microorganisms (see Sect. 9). These saprophytes or commensals are important for the maintenance of general health, for they retard invasion by pathogenic microorganisms [286].

If foreign pathogenic organisms reach the skin, an infection *may* occur. This depends on a variety of factors, such as the number and virulence of the foreign microorganisms, the state of the skin surface, and the state of the physiologic defense systems. This is discussed further in Sect. 9.

The disturbance of the normal microbial balance promotes diseases and infections of the skin. Excessive washing with alkali esters of higher fatty acids (soaps) or even infrequent washing in predisposed persons is sometimes sufficient to disturb the saprophytes either directly or indirectly (via changes on the skin surface). Certain soap additives can heighten this effect. Common modes of social behavior, certain hygienic habits, and numerous medications (cytostatics, glucocorticoids, hormones, and even antimicrobials) all contribute to the increase of microbial infections in man (details in Sects. 9 and 10).

Disregarding the deeper-seated pyodermas and tinea profunda, there are two main types of microbial changes on the skin surface: (1) microbial infections in the strict sense, and (2) secondary infections ("secondary invasions," "colonization") of inflamed skin lesions, usually of the eczematous type. In the latter case the invading organisms may be either bacteria (gram-positive cocci) or fungi.

In the case of bacteria, for example, a distinction can be made only on the basis of the *number* of organisms present. It is assumed that an *infection* in the strict sense exists if there are at least 10^6 organisms per cm^2 [166]. If the number of staphylococci (these are almost entirely *Staphylococcus aureus*) is less than $10^6/cm^2$, a *secondary infection* is present. This distinction is important in terms of therapeutic procedure. In the latter case, anti-inflammatory therapy (e. g., with glucocorticoids) is sufficient; as the inflammation clears, the normal skin saprophytes will return, displacing the foreign microorganisms. Antimicrobial agents are unnecessary.

From a clinical standpoint, there are no clear criteria for differentiating between infection in the strict sense and secondary infection. In most cases, therefore, glucocorticoid therapy is combined with the local application of an antimicrobial agent. Because a determination of pathogen resistance is too time-consuming, even though a substance is needed that is reliably effective against the infecting organism, a dilemma arises in an era when microbes (especially staphylococci) are highly resistant to antibiotics. Consequently, broad-spectrum antimicrobials are usually administered.

The situation is somewhat less complicated in the case of dermato*mycoses*. Classical mycoses (tinea) are comparable to the true pyodermas (impetigo, furuncles). However, various infections caused by yeast fungi ("levuroses") and diseases caused by molds exhibit some features of the secondary infections described above. The causative agent in such "opportunistic" mycoses is obscure. An example is intertriginous mycosis on sweat-macerated skin. In such cases the use of a broad-spectrum antimycotic (e. g., an imidazole derivative) is advised.

An example of a microbial infection of the mucous membranes is vaginitis. Impermeable underclothing, the improper use of vaginal sprays, the taking of oral contraceptives, and the rise of "promiscuity" and "permissiveness" contribute to the occurrence of vaginal infections. Moreover, the specific treatment of *one* type of infection (e. g., giving metronidazole for trichomonas vaginitis) may promote the development of a levurosis, usually candidal vaginitis (see Sect. 10.5), by disturbing the microbial balance. A further and too often neglected therapeutic (and diagnostic) problem is that of double and multiple infections. Under some circumstances several types of microorganisms may inhabit a single lesion, or various coexisting lesions may be caused by different pathogens. Broad-spectrum antimicrobials are of particular value in such cases, for they allow all lesions, regardless of whether they are caused wholly or partly by dermatophytes, yeasts, molds, or staphylococci, to be successfully treated with a single drug preparation.

1.3 Antimicrobial Drugs for Local Application

Numerous drugs have been used during the evolution of medical therapeutics for the local treatment of mycotic and bacterial lesions of the skin and mucous membranes. Only a few have stood the test. Of historical interest are the mercury salts known from Arabic medicine, "chlorinated soda" (hypochlorite), and tincture of iodine, introduced as an antiseptic in 1939. Phenol is also counted among the "classical" antiseptics used for many years. However, such antiseptics are generally ill suited for the treatment of microbial lesions, owing to their poor skin tolerance and toxic properties.

It was not until the 1940s that local therapy was enriched by the introduction of disinfectants. The following requirements were placed on disinfectants for local application: microbicidal action; good solubility and stability; resistance to inhibition by substances on the skin surface or by blood, serum, or pus; absence of absorption; low toxicity; low sensitization index; and absence of photosensitizing properties. Few of these requirements were adequately fulfilled, the main problem being low tolerance in the presence of inflammation. Moreover, the sudden eradication of microbes was not always favorable; it sometimes triggered local and even general flare-up reactions (overtreatment phenomena).

One of the principal phenol derivatives with an antiseptic action employed in local antimicrobial therapy is *hexachlorophene;* however, absorptive effects, especially in children, reduce the clinical usefulness of hexachlorophene [36, 87]. Among the cationic antiseptics, *chlorhexidine* has attained the greatest importance in external therapy. Chlorhexidine is only mildly toxic and is well tolerated by the mucous membranes, but its antimicrobial action is not too strong.

The efficacy of antiseptics depends on three factors: concentration of the drug, duration of action, and cell density. Antiseptics are adsorbed to the cytoplasmic membranes of bacteria and fungi. This results in a change in membrane permeability that allows the leakage of low-molecular compounds from the cell. These changes are still reversible in the initial stage, but later lead to the death of the cell.

Other dermatologically important disinfectants are the *invert soaps.* However, invert soaps which are well tolerated by the skin usually have low antimicrobial activity. The invert soaps are generally not well tolerated by the mucous membranes, which frequently leads to unpleasant irritations during therapeutic use.

The *acridine dyes* and *quinoline derivatives* are highly effective and are usually well tolerated. But frequent sensitization, absorptive effects and their staining properties greatly limit the use of these compounds [42, 89, 90, 191]. *Triphenylmethane dyes* are no longer used in topical antimicrobial therapy, mainly due to their tendency to stain the skin and clothing.

The next class of substances to be introduced in the local treatment of skin infections were the *sulfonamides.* Despite their good antibacterial activity, the use of sulfonamides in local therapy soon had to be abandoned due to frequent sensitization. Today the local application of sulfonamides is considered to be contraindicated.

The era of sulfonamides in local therapy was followed by the era of antibiotics. However, the *antibacterial* antibiotics, especially streptomycin and penicillin, proved to be strongly sensitizing when applied externally. As a result, few antibacterial antibiotics are still used today in local therapy. The foremost of these is neomycin (the neomycins), which is not absorbed and is unsuited for systemic use. (Oral administration is used to combat intestinal pathogens; parenteral administration of neomycin is contraindicated due to toxic effects.) Neomycins rarely lead to sensitization, but caution is advised in the treatment of leg ulcers.

As mentioned in Sect. 1.1, antibiotics which are administered systemically should not be applied locally. For this reason alone, the number of antibiotics available for local antibacterial therapy is quite limited.

The situation is different in the case of *antimycotic antibiotics*. With the exception of griseofulvin, which is active only against dermatophytes, the antimycotic antibiotics (mostly polyene compounds) are not absorbed by the skin and mucous membranes. They cannot be administered parenterally due to their high toxicity and low solubility. An exception is the amphotericin B-deoxycholic acid complex, which can be administered intravenously. The high incidence of adverse effects from such therapy is discussed in detail in Sect. 10.8.1. Most of the antimycotic antibiotics are used exclusively for the local treatment of mycoses of the skin and mucous membranes.

The most widely used antifungal agents have been nystatin (yellow, active only against yeasts and molds), natamycin (colorless, active against yeasts, molds, and dermatophytes), and variotin (active against dermatophytes, cryptococci, and blastomyces) [233]. Like nystatin and natamycin, variotin is a tetraene (chemical compound with four conjugated double bonds) but unlike them, it is not a macrolide antibiotic (macrolides contain a multimembered ring with an oxygen bridge). Follow-up studies have shown a surprisingly high rate of sensitization by variotin [199], whereas nystatin (three cases of allergy to date) and natamycin (no cases of allergy to date) possess practically no sensitizing properties, as revealed by the experiences of 20 years of clinical use.

The advantage of the antibiotics lies in their good tolerance. Their disadvantages are their narrow antimicrobial spectra, the rapid rise of resistance quotas to antibacterial antibiotics, and the increasing sensitization rates. Consequently, there is now a trend back to the broad-spectrum chemotherapeutic agents and disinfectants; halogenated organic compounds are again finding frequent application despite their sometimes weak action, and quinoline derivatives despite their sensitizing properties and yellow staining of skin and clothing. The imidazole derivatives are among the safest and most effective substances known for local antimicrobial therapy.

2 Broad-Spectrum Antimicrobials for Local Application

2.1 Preliminary Remarks

Broad-spectrum antimicrobials are substances which are active in low concentrations against a variety of pathogenic and facultatively pathogenic microorganisms. *Broad-spectrum antimycotics,* on the other hand, are drugs whose activity spectrum covers all three groups of fungi pathogenic to man (dermatophytes, yeasts, molds).

According to the above definition, a variety of broad-spectrum antimicrobials exist, in the form of numerous disinfectants. However, the requirements of local therapy call for a substance which is also satisfactorily tolerated by inflamed skin. This is essential for its complication-free therapeutic use.

Broad-spectrum antibiotics are antibiotics which are active against various bacterial *or* fungal strains. Thus, for example, chloramphenicol is included among the antibacterial broad-spectrum antibiotics, and natamycin among the antimycotic broad-spectrum antibiotics. However, there is no broad-spectrum antibiotic which is active against fungal *and* bacterial strains. This is understandable, considering the mechanism of action of antibiotics.

In different branches of medicine, antimicrobials with different spectra of activity are desired. In dermatology, for example, substances which are active against all fungal strains and gram-positive bacteria are the most important, while antimicrobials for gynecologic use should be active mainly against yeasts and trichomonads.

Broad-spectrum antimicrobials that are active against fungi, bacteria, and protozoa and that are also well tolerated when applied locally are found only in the large family of chemotherapeutic agents.

2.2 Disinfectants and Antiseptics

The main purpose of disinfectants and antiseptics is the disinfection of wounds, the sterilization of healthy skin areas (preoperatively), and the cleaning of surgical instruments. They must also be active sporicidally.

Today, disinfectants no longer have a place in the local treatment of skin or mucous membrane changes. They are still sometimes used adjunctively for cleaning purposes. Their disadvantages are their poor skin tolerance, their tendency to cause photosensitivity reactions, their sensitizing potential, and their tendency to stain. The activity spectrum of the disinfectants and antiseptics is broad, encompassing fungi, bacteria, and protozoa (see Sect. 2.1).

2.3 Antibiotics

Despite their generally excellent tolerance, antibiotics are becoming increasingly less important in the local treatment of skin and mucous membrane infections. The reasons for this, as mentioned earlier, are the increasing sensitization of the population [247, 248], and the rising resistance quotas of the main pathogens, especially bacteria [17, 124, 161, 196, 286]. The growing problem of antibiotic therapy in general is reflected in such phrases as "choosing the lesser evil" or "compromising between risks and possible therapeutic benefits" [159].

Antibiotics usually exhibit only a narrow spectrum of activity. They are active against certain bacterial strains *or* certain fungal strains. For example, nystatin is active against yeasts and molds, but not against dermatophytes; griseofulvin, on the other hand, is active only against dermatophytes. However, drugs with a broad activity spectrum are preferred in local therapy, because it is often difficult to make an exact diagnosis in such cases, and frequently neither the time nor the facilities are available for pathogen identification or susceptibility testing prior to treatment.

The disadvantage of a narrow spectrum is offset by using combinations of antibiotics. For example, neomycin and gramicidin have frequently been combined with nystatin in a single preparation, or natamycin with neomycin. But while such preparations exhibit broad activity against fungi and bacteria, they double the risk of sensitization and have been widely rejected for that reason (see Sect. 13.2). This problem of sensitization is avoided in the case of polyene antibiotics, but the use of "poly" prepations subjects the skin surface to an increased drug load.

2.4 Chemotherapeutic Agents

Only a few chemotherapeutic agents have proved effective against bacteria *and* fungi. The first group to be mentioned are the quinoline derivatives (see Sect. 13.3), 5-chloro-7-iodo-8-hydroxyquinoline (clioquinol) and 5,7-dichloro-2-methyl-8-hydroxyquinoline (chlorquinaldol) often give very good results in the local treatment of superficial microbial infections, despite sensitizations and other intolerances. Other quinoline derivatives have proved unsatisfactory due to their stronger sensitizing properties [91, 150, 191]. The same considerations apply for the quinoline fluorides such as hydroxyquinoline-silico-fluoride and quinoline-silico-fluoride. Caution is advised when applying clioquinol to large skin areas, due to the possibility of absorptive effects [89].

Another important agent is haloprogin (chemical name 3-iodo-2-2propynyl-2,4,5-trichlorophenyl ether or 2,4,5-trichlorophenyl-8-iodopropargyl ether), an antimicrobial with good local tolerance and a broad activity spectrum [285]. However, this substance has not been in use long enough for a final assessment to be made. In particular, the questions of its permeation, its bioavailability, and its activity under the oxygen tension in the skin have not yet been fully resolved [246]. The halogenated phenol derivatives (e. g., hexachlorophene, chlorhexidine, triclosan) are excellently tolerated by the skin and mucous membranes, but they lead to photosensitivity reactions, toxic absorptive effects, and sensitization. Their activity may be diminished by lipids on the skin surface [205]. Only a few data are available on the pyridone derivatives, e. g. ciclopirox (formula shown in Fig. 41). Ciclopirox is described as an antimycotic compound with broad spectrum of activity [66a]. Experimental studies revealed a surprisingly high penetration rate of ciclopirox into horny material [66].

Some antifungal compounds exhibit limited spectra, only. For example, tolnaftate, tolciclate, and pyrrolnitrin (3-chloro-4-[3-chloro-2-nitrophenyl]-pyrrol) [334] are active against dermatophytes but not against yeasts.

The imidazole derivatives are the latest development in the area of broad-spectrum antimicrobials. They are highly active against all fungi pathogenic to man. Clotrimazole, miconazole, and econazole are also active against gram-positive bacteria. From a clinical pharmacologic standpoint, the imidazole derivatives are superior to the substances previously mentioned (see Sect. 8).

2.5 Imidazole Derivatives with Antimicrobial Action

2.5.1 General

As early as 30 years ago, it was found that benzimidazole (Fig. 1) inhibits the growth of fungi and bacteria. This inhibitory action is abolished by the addition of the purine bases, adenine or guanine (structural formulas in Fig. 1). This finding led to the following hypothesis regarding the mode of action of benzimidazoles: *Benzimidazoles competitively inhibit the uptake of important metabolites into the cell and thus interfere with cell growth.*

It was then observed, about 20 years ago, that substituted benzimidazoles have stronger antimycotic properties, particularly when the substitution is in

8

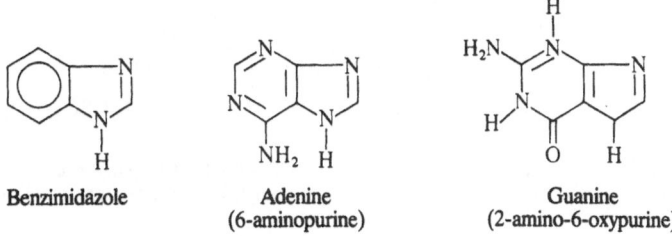

Benzimidazole   Adenine   Guanine
(6-aminopurine)   (2-amino-6-oxypurine)

Fig. 1. Structural formulas of benzimidazole, guanine, and adenine

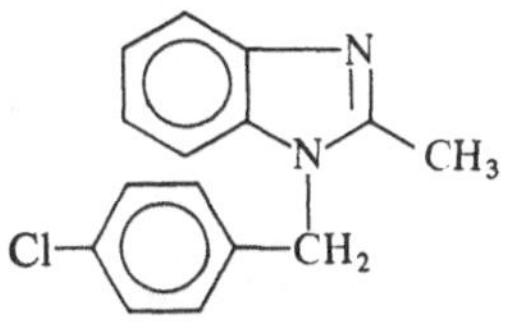

Fig. 2. Structural formula of chlormidazole (1-*p*-chlorobenzyl-2-methylbenzimidazole)

the 2-position [127]. Synthesis research and extensive series of tests led to the development of chlormidazole, chemical name 1-*p*-chlorobenzyl-2-methyl-benzimidazole (Fig. 2), an antifungal for local application [249].

Chlormidazole was the first *azole antimycotic* used in medicine. The azole antimycotics are distinguished by two structural properties: They contain an unsubstituted imidazole or triazole ring, and the rest of the molecule is linked by a nitrogen-carbon bridge. The azole antimycotics are active against all fungi pathogenic to man (they are broad-spectrum antimycotics) and exert a fungicidal action even in extremely low concentrations. They sometimes lead to enzyme induction in the macroorganism (clear species-dependence!), which results in an increasingly rapid breakdown in the liver on repeated use [215].

In the years that followed, numerous chemical modifications and substitutions in the benzimidazole molecule led to the development of important new drugs for human use. The orally administered antitrichomonal drugs metronidazole and tinidazole and the antihelmintic drugs niridazole, thiabendazole, and mebendazole are examples. The formulas of some imidazole derivatives for systemic therapy are shown in Fig. 3. The spectra of the major imidazole derivatives are given in simplified form in Table 1. Of the compounds mentioned here, only thiabendazole has attained importance in local therapy. Thiabendazole has proved highly effective against dermatophytoses when applied in the form of a cream or ethanol solution.

Of particular interest among the imidazole derivatives is levamisole, which has an immune-stimulating or immune-modulating action (formula in Fig. 3). Levamisole has been tried with varying success in the treatment of recurrent herpes infections (survey in [238]). Today this substance is primarily of onco-

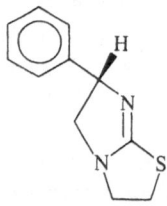

Metronidazole (1-β-
hydroxyethyl-2-methyl-
5-nitroimidazole)

Tinidazole (1-[2-(ethyl-sulfonyl)-
ethyl]-2-methyl-5-nitroimidazole)

Niridazole (1-(5-nitro-2-
thiazolyl)-imidazolidine-2-one)

Thiabendazole (2-(4′-thiazolyl)-
benzimidazole)

Mebendazole (methyl-5-(6)-benzoyl-2-
benzimidazole-carbamate)

Levamisole (L-2,3,5,6-tetrahydro-
6-phenylimidazole-(2,1b)-thiazole)

Fig. 3. Structural formulas of some therapeutically important imidazole derivatives

logical interest, however, despite adverse effects which may be considerable in
some instances. This point is mentioned here because miconazole (see [353])
and econazole were also thought to influence the immune system.

The latest developments from the series of imidazole derivatives are the
drugs clotrimazole, miconazole, isoconazole, and econazole, intended primarily
for local application, and ketoconazole, intended for oral use.

10

Table 1. Activity spectra of some systemically administered imidazole derivatives

Substance	Bacteria	Activity against Fungi	Protozoa	Helminths
Metronidazole Timorazole Tinidazole Ronidazole	Anaerobes Anaerobes Anaerobes Dysentric bacteria	– – – –	Trichomonads *Giardia* Trypanosomes Amoebas	– –
Thiabendazole	–	*Trichophyton* *Microsporum* *Aspergillus* (local application)	–	Nematodes (systemic)
Mebendazole	–	*Trichophyton* *Aspergillus*	–	Nematodes
Tetramisole Levamisole[a]	– –	– –	– –	Nematodes Nematodes
Niridazole	–	–	–	Schistosomes *Dracunculus*
Clotrimazole Miconazole[b] Isoconazole[b] Econazole[b] Ketoconazole	Gram-positives	Yeasts Molds *Trichophyton* *Microsporum*	Trichomonads Amoebas	–

[a] Immune stimulant!   [b] Nitrates are unsuited for systemic administration.

2.5.2 Chlormidazole

Chlormidazole (formula in Fig. 2) was the first imidazole derivative to achieve importance in the local treatment of mycoses. Chlormidazole is used in a concentration of 5% (cream, solution). It is exclusively suited for the external treatment of dermatomycoses in man and animals. Tests have shown minimum inhibitory concentrations of about 6.3 μg/ml for *Trichophyton,* 25 μg/ml for *Microsporum,* 156 μg/ml for *Candida albicans,* and 39 μg/ml for *Penicillium notatum* [249].

2.5.3 Clotrimazole

Clotrimazole (Fig. 4) is an imidazole derivative with a trityl structure (*bis*-phenyl-[2-chlorophenyl]-1-imidazolyl methane). Clotrimazole has demonstrated the best antimycotic activity out of the entire series of similarly active trityl imidazoles. Some trityl imidazoles have found application as plant fungicides.

Clotrimazole is effective against dermatophytes, yeasts, and molds. It is also active antibacterially. Its minimum inhibitory concentration for staphylococci ranges up to 50 μ/ml. Clotrimazole is active against amoebas *(Naegleria fowleri)* in concentrations of 1 μg/ml; against *Trichomonas vaginalis* its trichomonacidal concentration is 100 μg/ml. Clotrimazole is also active against *Toxoplasma.*

Numerous series of tests have been done to determine whether it is possible to increase the laboratory resistance of yeasts and other fungal strains to clotrimazole. In series of up to 22 passages *in vitro* over various culture media with increasing concentrations of clotrimazole, no enhancement of resistance could be achieved. This indicates that fungi undergo neither a one-step nor an oligo-step mutation in the presence of imidazole derivatives. This was confirmed by tests with the other antimicrobially active imidazole derivatives as well.

Clotrimazole is also active systemically. It is absorbed when administered orally (detection of blood levels). For a review on clotrimazole, cf. [266].

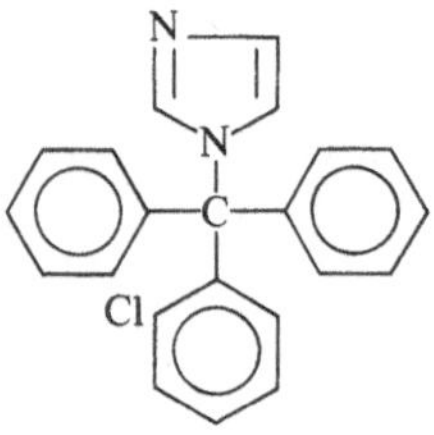

Fig. 4. The structural formula of clotrimazole (bis-phenyl-[2-chlorophenyl-1-imidazolyl]-methane)

2.5.4 Miconazole and Isoconazole

With the development of the imidazole derivative miconazole (Fig. 5), another substance was introduced into local therapy that can be classified as a broad-spectrum antimycotic on the one hand, and is active against gram-positive bacteria on the other. This is an extremely important property, for long-standing fungal infections are commonly contaminated by large numbers of staphylococci [149]. These bacteria play a pathogenic role in the perpetuation of the lesion. Drugs with antimycotic *and* antibacterial activity lead to healing more quickly than simple antimycotics. For a review on miconazole, cf. [265].

Like clotrimazole, miconazole is absorbed when administered orally; therapeutic serum levels can be achieved in humans (see Sects. 6.3 and 11). Miconazole can also be administered intravenously. Its efficacy when applied systemically has been confirmed in experiments on various animal species [59, 163, 165, 271]. For further details, see Sect. 5.2.

Isoconazole is an isomer of miconazole. The structural formula of miconazole is 1-2,4-dichloro-β-(2,4-dichlorobenzyloxy)-phenethylimidazole; the formula for isoconazole is 1-2,4-dichloro-ß-(2,6-dichlorobenzyloxy)-phenethylimidazole. The antimicrobial activity of isoconazole largely corresponds to that of miconazole.

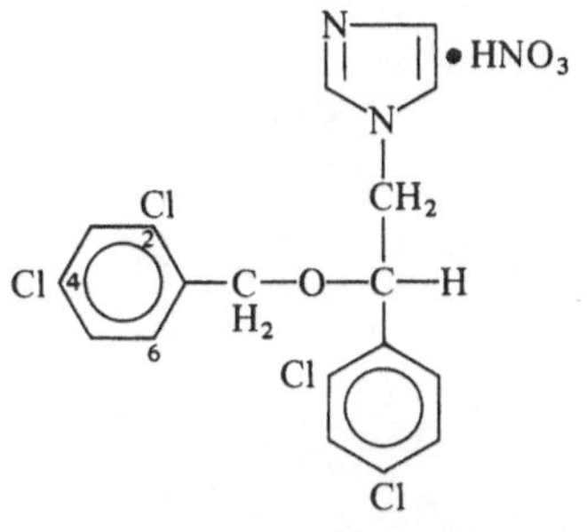

Miconazole nitrate (1-{2-(2,4-dichloro-phenyl)-2-[(2,4-dichlorophenyl)-methoxy]-ethyl}-1H-imidazole nitrate)

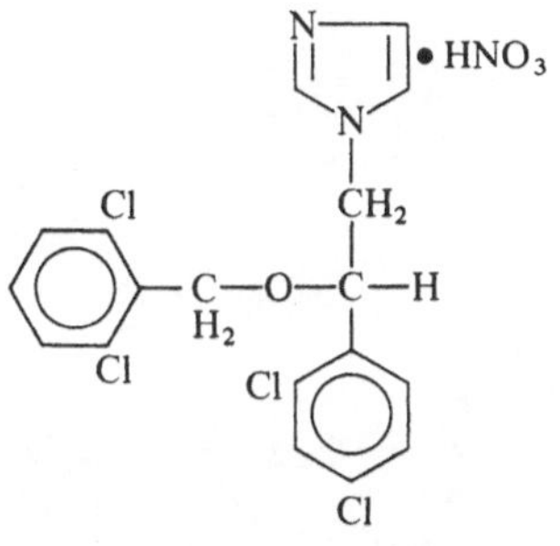

Isoconazole nitrate (1-{2-(2,4-dichloro-phenyl)-2-[(2,6-dichlorophenyl)-methoxy]-ethyl}-1H-imidazole nitrate)

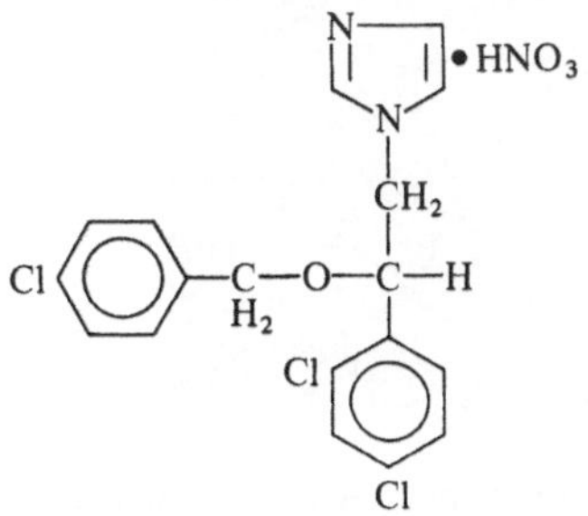

Econazole nitrate (1-[2-(2,4-dichlorophenyl)-2-(4-chlorobenzyloxy)-ethyl]-imidazole nitrate)

Fig. 5. The structural formulas of miconazole nitrate, isoconazole nitrate and econazole nitrate

2.5.5 Econazole

The econazole molecule contains a doubly chlorinated aromatic ring. In contrast to miconazole, the second aromatic ring carries only *one* chlorine atom (structural formula in Fig. 5). The spectrum of activity of econazole is extraordinarily similar to that of miconazole, although it possesses a somewhat higher antimicrobial activity (see below), which is probably due at least in part to its modified (improved in an antimicrobial or galenic sense) physical properties (lower molecular weight, "smaller" molecule). Like other imidazole derivatives, econazole acts on the surface of the fungal cells (Fig. 6 and 7).

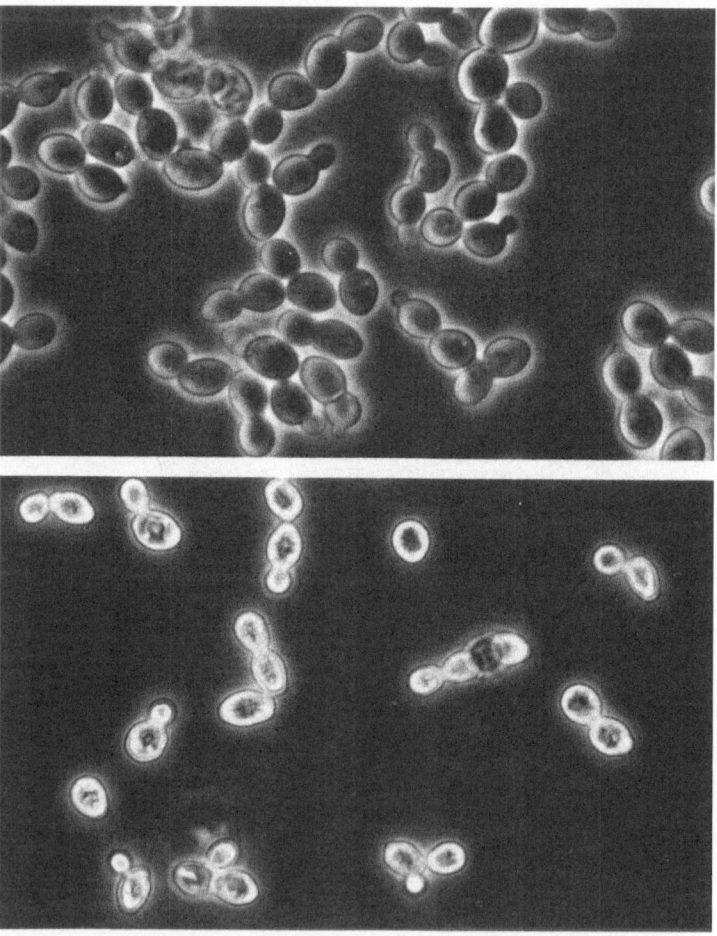

Fig. 6. Effect of econazole on *Candida albicans* as shown by phase-contrast microscopy. *Top:* 35-h-old control culture untreated with econazole. *Bottom:* 24 h after treatment with 10 µg/ml econazole, dense deposits are observed within the cells. The cells are no longer capable of reproduction

Econazole, like miconazole, is used in the form of its nitrate when applied locally. Owing to its somewhat higher activity, econazole nitrate is used in 1% preparations; miconazole nitrate is used at 2% concentration in ordinary preparations (exception: tincture). For a review on econzale, cf. [118].

Both econazole and miconazole can be used in the treatment of systemic mycoses. They are administered either in the form of gastric-acid-resistant capsules or by intravenous injection or infusion. In this case the pure base, rather than the nitrate, is used. Econazole is considered one of the best external broad-spectrum antimycotic agents. One the one hand, it possesses a high and broad antimicrobial activity (active against all fungi pathogenic to man and

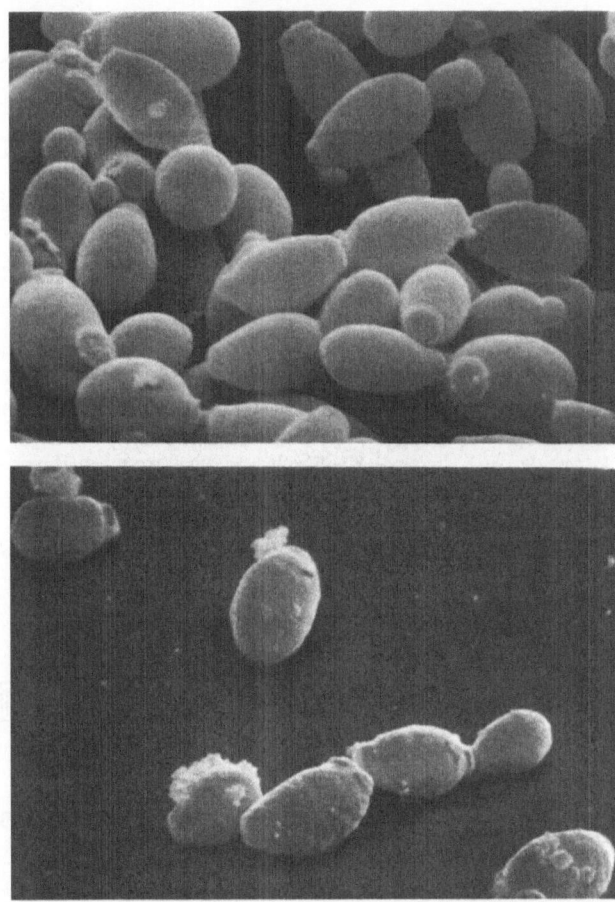

Fig. 7. Scanning electron micrograph of *Candida albicans*. Control cells *(top)* and yeasts after 4 h exposure to econazole in a concentration of 50 µg/ml *(bottom)*. The cell surface is irregular in shape and shows protrusions of material from numerous ruptures (after [6, 7])

15

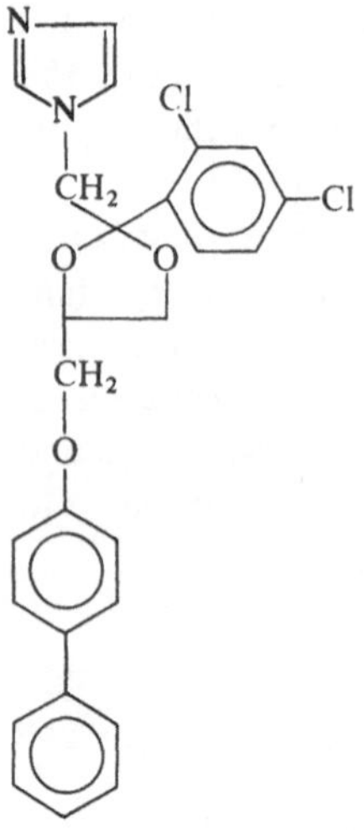

R-34000 (Parent compound of ketoconazole)

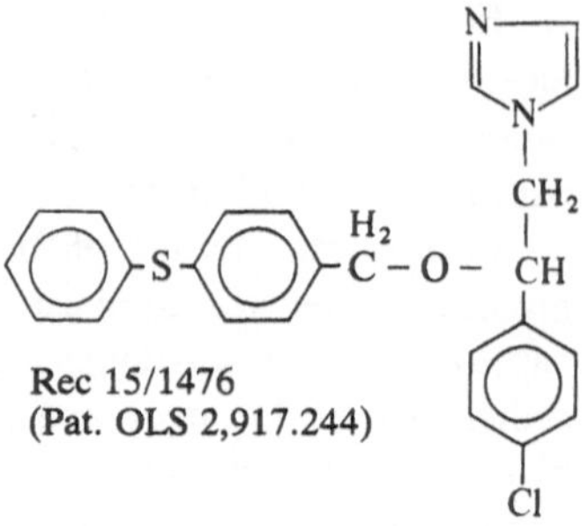

Rec 15/1476
(Pat. OLS 2,917.244)

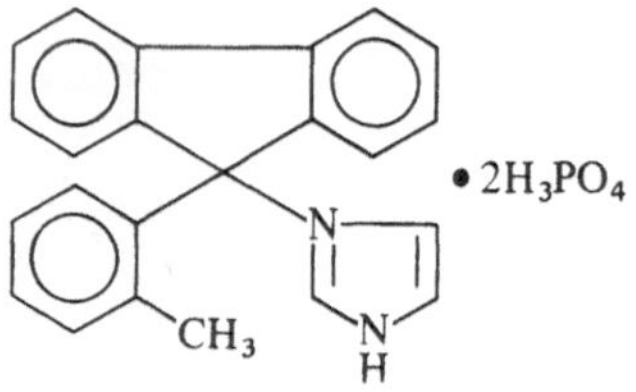

$\cdot 2H_3PO_4$

BAY h 4364

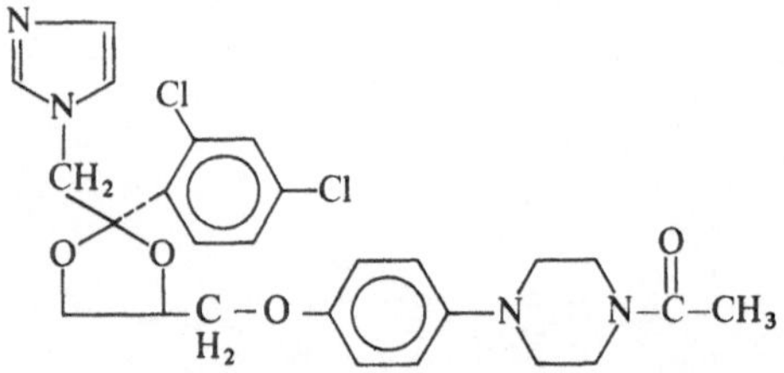

Ketoconazole, (*cis*-1-acetyl-4-[4-[[2-(2,4-dichlorophenyl)-2-
(1 *H*-imidazole-1-ylmethyl)-1,3-dioxolan-4-yl]methoxy]phenyl] piperazine)

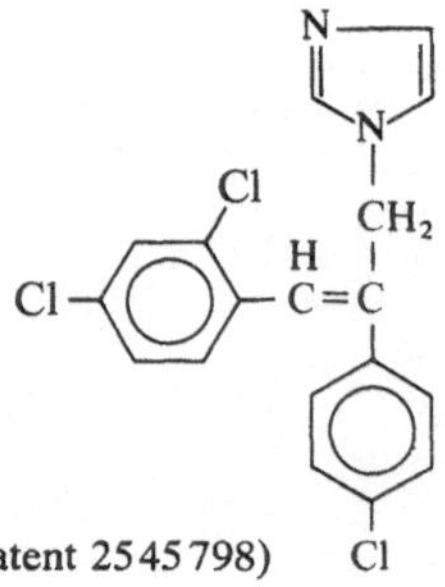

N⁻148/76
(German patent 25 45 798)

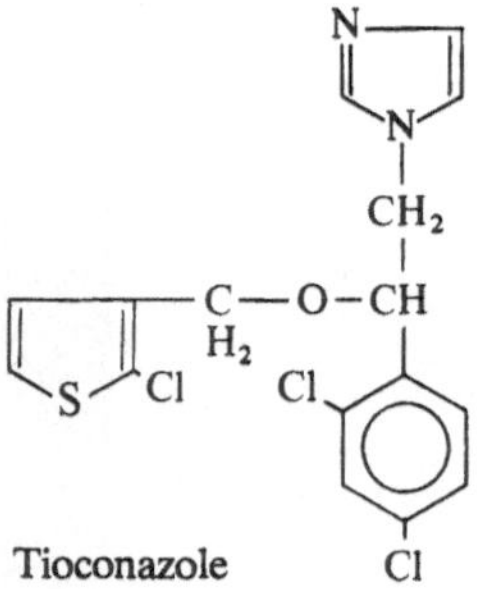

Tioconazole

Fig. 8. The structural formulas of R-34000 [cis-biphenyl-4-yloxymethyl-2-(2,4-dichloro-phenyl)-1,3-dioxolane-2-yl-methyl imidazole (M = 481)], of ketoconazole (M = 531), of BAY h 4364 (M = 519), of N-148/76 (trans-1-(2,4-dichlorophenyl)-2-(4-chlorophe-nyl)-3-(imidazolyl-1)-propen-1-hydrochloride (M = 400), of Rec 15/1476 (M = 518), and of tioconazole (M = 369)

against gram-positive bacteria); and on the other, econazole best satisfies the requirements of the clinical pharmacologist. Good penetration is obtained during external use. It is well tolerated, and antimicrobial concentrations are reliably achieved even in deeper skin layers (see Sect. 8).

2.5.6 Ketoconazole

Ketoconazole (R 41400), the formula of which is shown in Fig. 8, exhibits about the same spectrum of antimicrobial activity as miconazole. In some *in vitro* models, e. g., in the manometric investigations of resting *Saccharomyces cerevisiae* (personal investigations, unpublished) ketoconazole showed less activity; in some others, e. g., on *Candida albicans* grown in media which commonly are used for the cultivation of mammalian cells, it was found to be more potent [41, 67].

The striking difference, however, from all other imidazole derivatives known so far is the excellent absorption upon oral administration. One tablet of 200 mg/ketoconazole produces plasma levels in human volunteers of about 5 µg/ml, which is well above the minimal inhibitory concentration of most fungi pathogenic to man. Although ketoconazole is still in the stage of clinical evaluation, the results collected so far seem most promising. Ketoconazole was successfully used in coccidiodomycosis, paracoccidiodomycosis, histoplasmosis, candidosis (e. g., in vaginal candidosis 2 × 200 mg/day for 3 days), onychomycosis, and tinea. Dermatologists reported good results with oral ketoconazole in dermatomycoses and onychomycoses; adverse effects were absent [44 a, 107 a]. Those facts were confirmed by personal experiences.

2.5.7 Assessment of Imidazole Derivatives

The family of imidazole derivatives has substantially enriched the area of local antimycotic therapy. According to initial results, they certainly bring significant improvements to the treatment of systemic mycoses as well. A final assessment is not yet possible, however.

Other derivatives, such as a dioxolane imidazole or a clotrimazole derivative (formulas given in Fig. 8) have proved effective when given orally or have exhibited better pharmacokinetics than clotrimazole [162, 215]. According to the data compiled until now, ketoconazole will be the drug of choice for the oral treatment of fungal infections of man (cf. Sect. 2. 5. 6). N-148/76, (formula shown in Fig. 8), another new imidazole antifungal, which still is in the process of experimental and pharmacological evaluation, seems quite promising for topical and systemic treatment, too. Tioconazole (Fig. 8), a compound with a similar structure as miconazole, is four times more active against Candida spp. than miconazole *in vitro* [356]. Today, *clinical* data on tioconazole are not yet available. One may assume that more and more imidazole derivatives (example: Rec 15/1476, formula in Fig. 8) will be introduced as antifungals in medical therapy in the not too distant future. – In closing this chapter, a short assessment will be given of the three most important imidazole derivatives with antifungal action for *topical* use.

Chlormidazole, the first imidazole derivative used against dermatomycoses, exhibits a comparatively weaker antimycotic activity and was introduced in the form of 5% preparations. It is inactive against bacteria. *Clotrimazole* has developed in the last decade into an important drug for the local treatment of dermatologic and gynecologic mycoses. The broad spectrum of clotrimazole covers all the fungi pathogenic to man, as well as gram-positive bacteria.

Miconazole and *econazole* also exhibit a very broad spectrum of activity. These drugs are active against all fungi pathogenic to man and against gram-positive bacteria; they protect against overgrowth of trichomonads in the same way as clotrimazole. Thus, only gram-negative organisms are missing from their activity spectrum; but these organisms are of only minor importance in superficial infections of the skin and mucous membranes (see Sect. 9).

The imidazole derivatives are superior to all other antimycotics in terms of broadness of spectrum and level of overall activity. Differences found *in vitro* within the group of imidazole derivatives can often be attributed to experimental conditions [111].

It is surprising at first sight that two substances as similar chemically as miconazole and econazole, which differ by only one chlorine atom, should exhibit such quantitatively different antimicrobial activities. For example, econazole nitrate is applied locally in a 1% concentration, while miconazole is used in the form of 2% preparations. It must be realized, however, that even slight changes in molecular structure (10% difference in molecular weight!) can alter the penetration of the drug. Furthermore, lipophilicity must be taken into account (log p value of econazole 3.85, of miconazole 5.87). Under some circumstances such factors play an important role in skin penetration, in the release of the drug from the preparation (bioavailability), and in the development of the antimicrobial action.

Because of its great significance, one of the most important of the locally applied broad-spectrum antimycotics and broad-spectrum antimicrobials, econazole nitrate, will be discussed in detail in the next section as an example of the modern imidazole derivatives.

3 Econazole

3.1 General

Based on the results of experimental and clinical tests to date, econazole nitrate is excellent for the local treatment of fungal infections of the skin and mucous membranes. It is superior in many ways to other antifungal compounds in terms of efficacy and tolerance. Econazole was synthesized about 10 years ago in the laboratories of Janssen in Beerse, Belgium. Further research and development to the point of clinical application were carried out by Cilag-Chemie in Schaffhausen, Switzerland. Miconazole and ketoconazole were also synthesized by Janssen, while clotrimazole was developed by Bayer.

3.2 Chemical Structure

Econazole is the nontrademarked international name (Rec. I. N. N.) of the World Health Organization for 1-[2-(2,4-dichlorophenyl)-2-(4-chlorobenzyl-oxy)-ethyl]-imidazole nitrate. The structural formula of econazole is shown in Fig. 5. Its empirical formula is $C_{18}H_{15}Cl_3N_2O \cdot HNO_3$.

The molecular weight of econazole base is 381.68. The molecular weight of econazole nitrate is 444.70.

3.3 Physical Properties

Econazole is a white, odorless, amorphous or microcrystalline powder with a melting point between 160° and 168 °C. Its *ultraviolet absorption* maxima are at 218, 266, 272, and 280 nm; its minima are at 247, 269, and 278 nm (solvent: 90% isopropanol and 10% 0.1 mol/liter HCl).

The *stability* of econazole is excellent in dissolved and undissolved form in contrast to other antifungal drugs even at room temperature [102]. Econazole is nonhygroscopic. Its *solubility* in water is slight (maximum 0.05%). Econazole nitrate shows good solubility in methanol and dimethyl formamide.

For purity testing, it is important that the chemical structure of econazole can be verified according to standard procedures by the following methods: ultraviolet absorption, infrared absorption, NMR absorption, and mass-spectrographic analysis. Thin-film chromatography and gas chromatography are also suitable for identification and determination of plasma levels [47]. The pK_a value of econazole nitrate lies at pH 4.8. Its buffer capacity is greatest in this range. Econazole nitrate is present as a cation only at a more acidic pH, at which point its membrane penetration, absorption, and antimicrobial activity are reduced. This point is of particular importance during therapeutic use on the outer skin (acid film!) and on the vaginal epithelium (see below). The physical properties of a substance have a strong influence on its *therapeutic applicability.* This is true of topical agents as well. Bioavailability is determined by interrelationships between the drug, the vehicle or solvent, and the (diseased) skin surface. Slight changes in physical properties often have marked effects on bioavailability.

Econazole nitrate exhibits no polymeric forms; this precludes rearrangements of its crystalline structure. Econazole nitrate undergoes no decomposition or inactivation under normal drug storage conditions in the galenic preparations currently used. In many topical preparations, 50% of the econazole nitrate is present in dissolved form and 50% in solid form; in the same preparations, only about 10% of the miconazole nitrate is dissolved, and 90% is in solid form. But the bioavailability of a drug, and thus its clinical efficacy, is greatly enhanced when it is in dissolved form.

For systemic application, econazole is tested in the form of gastric-acid-resistant capsules and injection solutions. For local application, econazole nitrate is available in the form of a cream, a powder, and a lotion, as well as a vaginal cream and as vaginal suppositories.

3.4 Antimicrobial Spectrum

3.4.1 Antifungal Activity

When econazole nitrate is tested for its fungicidal properties, the same points must be considered as with all other azole antimycotics: the action is dependent on the medium, especially in the presence of certain lipids; on the number of microorganisms present, suggesting that the drug binds to cell surfaces; and on the presence of oxygen. The azole antimycotics exhibit higher activities in the blood and tissues, owing to the oxygen tension there, than under atmospheric conditions. This contrasts with the behavior of other antimycotics such as haloprogin [215].

The concentrations of azole antimycotics which *inhibit growth* are approximately 100 times higher than the concentrations which *inhibit cell division* in the same fungus strain. The minimum inhibitory concentrations of econazole for the principal *dermatophytes* are between 0.1 and 1 µg/ml. These values make econazole decidedly superior to the formerly most active standard substance, tolnaftate. The fungistatic activities of econazole and tolnaftate against dermatophytes are compared in Table 2 [309]. The values presented here have been confirmed by other investigators employing various other methods. (While the determination of *in vitro* activity must be the first step in testing a new antimicrobial agent, the results of the various tests for clinical efficacy should not be overrated.)

The inhibitory concentrations of econazole for various medically relevant yeasts and yeastlike organisms range from 10 to 100 µg/ml (complete inhibi-

Table 2. Comparison of the fungistatic activity of econazole (E) and tolnaftate (T) for dermatophytes (reading after 14 days, after [309])

Fungus strain	C	CS	1000 µg/ml		100 µg/ml		10 µg/ml		1 µg/ml		0.1 µg/ml		0.01 µg/ml		0.001 µg/ml	
			E	T	E	T	E	T	E	T	E	T	E	T	E	T
Microsporum canis (RV 14314)	●	●	○	○	○	○	○	○	○	◕	○	◔	◔	●	◔	●
Microsporum canis (RV 16465)	●	●	○	○	○	○	○	◕	○	◑	◕	●	◔	●	◔	●
Microsporum audouini	●	●	○	○	○	◕	○	◕	○	◑	◕	◔	◔	●	●	●
Trichophyton mentagrophytes (RV 14013)	●	●	○	○	○	○	○	○	○	◕	○	○	○	◔	◕	●
Trichophyton mentagrophytes (RV 14126)	●	●	○	○	○	○	○	○	○	◕	○	◑	○	◔	◕	●
Trichophyton rubrum (RV 14155)	●	●	○	○	○	○	○	○	○	○	○	○	◕	◑	◑	●
Trichophyton rubrum (RV 15715)	●	●	○	○	○	○	○	○	○	○	◕	○	◑	◑	◔	●
Trichophyton tonsurans	●	●	○	○	○	○	○	○	○	◑	○	◔	◔	●	●	●
Trichophyton verrucosum	●	●	○	○	○	○	○	○	○	○	○	◔	◕	●	●	●
Trichophyton interdigitale	●	●	○	○	○	◕	○	◕	○	◕	◕	◔	●	●	◔	●
Trichophyton ferrugineum	●	●	○	○	○	◕	○	◕	○	◕	◕	◑	●	●	◔	●
Langeronia soudanensis	●	●	○	○	○	○	○	○	○	◕	◕	◔	◑	◔	●	●
Trichophyton violaceum	●	●	○	○	○	○	○	○	○	◑	○	◔	◑	◔	●	●
Epidermophyton floccosum	●	●	○	○	○	○	○	○	○	○	○	◕	○	●	●	●
Microsporum gypseum	●	●	○	○	○	◕	○	◕	○	◕	◕	●	●	●	●	●

C = control, CS = control solvent (ethanol).
○ = complete inhibition
◕ = partial inhibition (about 75%)
◑ = partial inhibition (about 50%)
◔ = partial inhibition (about 25%)
● = no inhibition

Table 3. Comparison of the fungistatic activity of econazole and nystatin for various yeasts (3 U nystatin/ml = 1 µg/ml; symbols as in Table 2)

Fungus strain	Econazole (µg/ml)									Nystatin (µg/ml)					
	C	CS	1000	100	10	1	0.1	0.01	0.001	1666	333	33	3.3	0.3	0.03
Saccharomyces cerevisiae	●	●	○	○	◐	●	●	●	●	○	○	○	◐	●	●
Torulopsis glabrata	●	●	○	○	◐	◐	●	●	●	○	○	◐	◐	●	●
Cryptococcus neoformans	●	●	○	○	○	◐	●	●	●	○	○	○	◐	●	●
Candida tropicalis	●	●	○	○	◐	◐	●	●	●	○	○	◐	◐	●	●
Candida albicans (RV 4688)	●	●	○	○	●	●	●	●	●	○	○	○	◐	●	●
Candida albicans (RV 1995 L)	●	●			◐	●	●	●	●	○	○	○	◐	●	●
Candida krusei	●	●	○	○	◐	◐	●	●	●	○	○	○	●	●	●
Candida paropsilosis	●	●	○	○	○	●	●	●	●	○	○	◐	◐	●	●
Candida stellatoidea	●	●	○	○	○	◐	●	●	●	○	○	○	◐	●	●
Candida pseudotropicalis	●	●	○	○	○	◐	◑	◐	●	○	○	◐	●	●	●
Trichosporon cutaneum	●	◐	○	○	○	◐	◑	●	●	○	○	○	◐	●	●
Rhodotorula sp.	●		○	○	◐	●	●	●	●	○	○	○	●	●	●

C = control, CS = control solvent (ethanol).

tion of growth). When compared with nystatin, a tetraene antibiotic taken as a positive reference substance in terms of antimicrobial activity against yeasts, econazole was found to be at least its equal: Econazole was clearly more effective than nystatin against 12 yeasts tested (Table 3) [309]. When calculated on a moles-per-liter basis, the activity of econazole decreased in comparison with nystatin (molecular weight 950).

Table 4 shows the fungistatic activity of econazole against various molds and causative organisms of systemic mycoses. With the exception of four species, growth inhibition was achieved at concentration of only 1 μg/ml. Practically no differences are found between econazole and econazole nitrate in the usual microbiologic activity measurements [271].

Other authors have determined the fungistatic inhibitory concentrations of econazole nitrate in serial dilution tests on Sabouraud's glucose agar. Different values were obtained, depending on the time of the reading. In the *Candida* species, concentrations of only 0.36 μg/ml had a marked inhibitory effect (reading after 24 h); *Mucor mucedo* exhibited the lowest sensitivity to the drug (Table 5).

The high activity of econazole nitrate against yeasts was also confirmed in the Warburg test (manometric measurement of oxygen consumption). Two techniques were employed in the test: measurement of the oxygen consumption of resting organisms, and measurement of the oxygen consumption of proliferating organisms. In the first case, conditions are somewhat similar to those in secondary infections (saprophytes or facultatively pathogenic organisms). The proliferation tests, on the other hand, correspond roughly to the conditions of fungus metabolism during infection. Figure 9 shows the dose-response curve of econazole nitrate for resting *Saccharomyces cerevisiae* and for resting *Candida albicans*. As Fig. 9 indicates, econazole nitrate causes a greater inhibition of oxygen consumption in *Candida albicans* than in *Saccharomyces cerevisiae*. The advantage of the Warburg test lies in the fact that even relatively poorly soluble substances can be tested over a wide range of concentrations by selecting a suitable medium.

Investigations with a Coulter counter confirm the high activity of imidazole derivatives against *Candida albicans:* antimycotic effects are produced by concentrations between 0.1 and 0.06 fmol/cell [48]. The onset of antimycotic action occurred relatively late in some microbiologic tests: measurements of action kinetics by turbidimetric methods showed an onset of action after 105 min for the imidazole derivatives; for the polyene antibiotics nystatin, natamycin and amphotericin B, antimycotic action was clearly demonstrable after only 25 min [22]. The situation is different in Warburg tests on resting organisms: here the antimycotic action (inhibition of oxygen consumption by econazole nitrate) begins within 20 min [242], while equal concentrations of nystatin or natamycin sometimes take up to 1 h to cause a significant decrease in oxygen consumption [233].

Recently, a new test with high clinical relevance was introduced: the contact test [107]. Scales with the infecting organisms were put in contact with test

Table 4. Fungistatic activity of econazole against various saprophytic fungi and fungi pathogenic to man, animals, and plants (after [309]; symbols as in Table 2)

Fungus strain	Econazole		1000 μg/ml	100 μg/ml	10 μg/ml	1 μg/ml	0.1 μg/ml	0.01 μg/ml	0.001 μg/ml
	C	CS							
Absidia ramosa	●	●	○	○	◐	◐			
Mucor sp.	●	●	○	○	○	●			
Basidiobolus meristosporus	●	●	○	○	◐	◐			
Rhizopus sp.	●	●	○	○	○	●			
Entomophthora coronata	●	◐	○	○	◐	●			
Mortierella sp.	●	●	○	◐	○	●			
Madurella mycetomi[b]	●	●	○	○	○	○	○	●	●
Streptomyces somaliensis	●	●	○	○	○	○	●	●	●
Streptomyces madurae[b]	●	◐	○	○	○	○	●	●	●
Streptomyces pelletieri[b]	●	●	○	○	○	○	◐	●	●
Nocardia asteroides	●	●	○	○	○	○	●	●	●
Nocardia brasiliensis	●	◐	○	○	○	◐	●	●	●
Blastomyces dermatitidis (A 641)	●	◐	○	○	○	○	◐	●	● MP
Blastomyces brasiliensis[b]	●	○	○	○	○	○	○	○	◐ MP
Histoplasma capsulatum	●	●	○	○	○	○	○	○	● MP
Blastomyces dermatitidis (RV 15455)	●	◐	○	○	○	○	◐	◐	● BP
Blastomyces dermatitidis (RV 15455)	●	◐	○	○	○	○	○	◐	◐ BP
Blastomyces dermatitis (A 641)	●	◐	○	○	○	○	○	◐	●
Aspergillus fumigatus	●	●	○	○	○	○	◐	●	●
Aspergillus flavus	●	●	○	○	○	○	◐	●	●
Aspergillus nidulans	●	◐	○	○	○	○	◐	◐	●

Aspergillus niger
Geotrichum candidum
Penicillium notatum
Sporothrix schenckii I
Sporothrix schenckii II
Allescheria boydii
Madurella grisea
Alternaria sp.
Fusarium sp.
Saprolegnia sp.
Aureobasidium pullulans
Scopulariopsis brevicaulis
Cephalosporium recifei[a]
Cladosporium wernecki[a]
Cladosporium trichoides[b]
Phialophora verrucosa
Phialophora pedrosoi[b]

C = control, CS = control solvent (ethanol). MP = mycelial phase, BP = budding phase. Reading after 2 weeks.
[a]Reading after 3 weeks.
[b]Reading after 4 weeks.

Table 5. Fungistatic activity of econazole nitrate in the serial dilution test (Sabouraud glucose agar)

Fungus strains tested		MIC [µg/ml]		
Dermatophytes		6 Days	9 Days	14 Days
. *Epidermophyton floccosum*	A 3004	3.12	3.12	6.25
. *Microsporum audouinii*	No 940 IP	3.12	50	50
. *Microsporum canis*	A 325	1.56	3.12	25
. *Trichophyton interdigitale*	No 428 IP	12.50	25	25
. *Trichophyton mentagrophytes*	No 877 IP	12.50	12.50	25
. *Trichophyton rubrum*	A 290	6.25	12.50	12.50
. *Trichophyton tonsurans*	A 4530	1.56	25	25
. *Trichosporon cutaneum*	A 350	12.50	25	50
Yeasts and yeastlike organisms		24 h	48 h	7 Days
. *Candida albicans*	No 3153 serotype A	0.36	1.56	12.50
. *Candida albicans*	No 4560 serotype A	0.36	6.25	25
. *Candida albicans*	No 3156 serotype B	0.36	1.56	12.50
. *Candida tropicals*	No 857 §	0.36	1.56	12.50
. *Candida parakrusei*	No 45 IP	0.36	6.25	25
. *Cryptococcus neoformans*	No 526	0.36	1.56	6.25
. *Torulopsis glabrata*	No 810 IP	0.36	6.25	12.50
. *Saccharomyces cerevisiae*	0.36	3.12	12.50	
Dimorphous fungi		6 Days	9 Days	14 Days
. *Aspergillus niger*	A 184	6.25	25	50
. *Aspergillus fumigatus*	A 193	3.12	12.50	12.50
. *Blastomyces dermatitidis*	No 60 IP	0.36	3.12	3.12
. *Histoplasma capsulatum*	No 1052 IP	1.56	3.12	3.12
. *Madurella mycetomi*	No 582 IP	0.78	3.12	3.12
. *Mucor mucedo*	A 56	12.50	50	100
. *Nocardia asteroides*	A 73	1.56	1.56	3.12
. *Penicillium notatum*	A 2430	0.78	1.56	6.25
. *Sporotrichum schenckii*	No 245 IP	12.50	50	50

substances for different periods of time. Afterwards the scales were inoculated into test tubes. After 3–6 min contact, preparations with 1% econazole nitrate killed all microbes; no fungi could be grown in the test tubes.

3.4.2 Antibacterial Activity

Like clotrimazole, miconazole and econazole have demonstrated an antibacterial activity, but only against gram-positive organisms. Serial dilution tests in two different media were done to determine the bactericidal (reading after 7 days) and bacteriostatic (reading after 2 days) activities of econazole. The bactericidal and bacteriostatic activity of econazole against gram-positive bacteria (staphylococci, streptococci) correspond roughly to the activity of benzyl penicillin (Table 6). Beyond a concentration of 10 µg/ml, econazole was com-

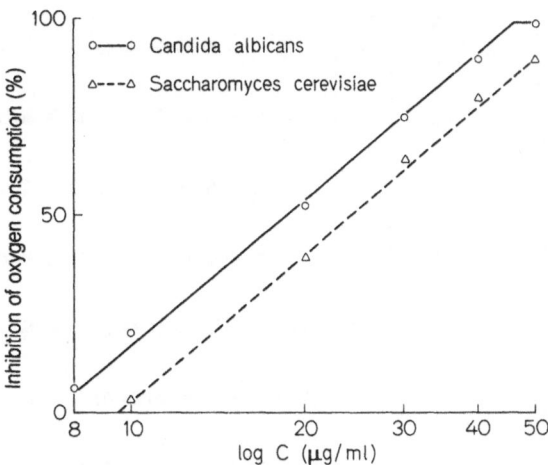

Fig. 9. Dose-response curve of econazole nitrate on resting *Saccharomyces cerevisiae* and resting *Candida albicans*. Warburg tests; medium: Ringer glucose with 3.3% dimethyl formamide; data in % inhibition of oxygen consumption relative to the control (solvent). Duration of test: 60 min, Oxygen consumation 124 ± 17 μl/h and 92 ± 8 μl/h, resp.

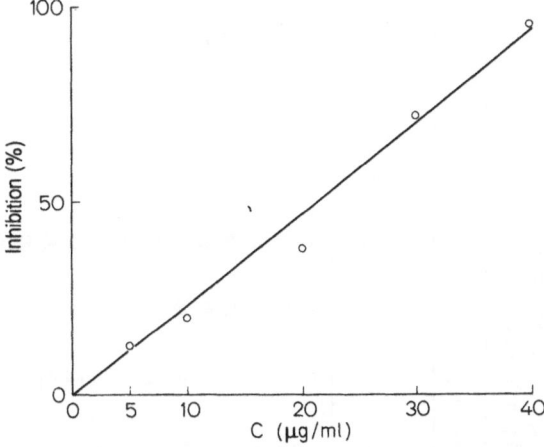

Fig. 10. Dose-response curve of econazole nitrate on resting *Staphylococcus aureus haemolyticus*. Medium: Ringer glucose with 3.3% dimethyl formamide. Inhibitory effect given in % of control; oxygen consumption in the controls = 57 ± 9 μl/h

pletely bactericidal and bacteriostatic in the gram-positive organisms tested. Econazole was ineffective against gram-negative bacteria [309], with the exception of bacteroides [340].

The effectiveness of econazole against gram-positive bacteria was repeatedly confirmed in further series of experiments. In the serial dilution test, the limits of bacteriostatic activity are often surprisingly low — between 0.36 and

Table 6. Comparison of the bacteriostatic and bactericidal activity of econazole (E) and sodium benzylpenicillin (P). Media: phenylsulfalein dextrose (D), tryptose broth (T), after [309] (symbols as in Table 2)

Reading after 48 h (bacteriostatic activity)

		C	CS	1000 µg/ml E	1000 µg/ml P	100 µg/ml E	100 µg/ml P	10 µg/ml E	10 µg/ml P	1 µg/ml E	1 µg/ml P	0.1 µg/ml E	0.1 µg/ml P	0.01 µg/ml E	0.01 µg/ml P
Erysipelothrix insidiosa	D	●	●	○		○	○	○	○	○	○	○	○	○	●
	T	●	●			○	○	○	○	○	○	○	○	●	●
Staphylococcus haemolyticus	D	●	●	○		○	○	○	○	○	○	○	○	●	●
	T	●	●			○	○	○	○	○	○	●	○	●	●
Staphylococcus aureus (B 2198)	D	●	●	○		○	○	○	●	●	●	●	●	●	●
	T	●	●			○	○	○	●	○	●	●	●	●	●
Staphylococcus aureus (B 1574)	D	●	●	○		○	○	○	●	●	●	●	●	●	●
	T	●	●			○	○	○	●	●	●	●	●	●	●
Streptococcus pyogenes	D	●	●	○		○	●	○	○	●	●	●	●	○	○
	T	●	●			○	○	○	○	●	○	●	●	○	○
Streptococcus faecalis	D	●	●	○		○	○	○	○	●	●	●	○	●	●
	T	●	●			○	○	○	○	●	●	●	●	●	●
Bacillus subtilis	D	●	●	○		○	○	○	○	●	○	●	○	●	●
	T	●	●			○	○	○	○	●	○	●	●	●	●
Bacillus anthracis	D	●	●	○		○	○	○	○	○	○	●	○	●	○
	T	●	●			○	○	○	○	●	○	●	●	●	●
Erysipelothrix insidiosa	D	●	●	○		○	○	○	○	○	○	○	○	●	●
	T	●	●			○	○	○	○	○	○	○	○	●	●
Staphylococcus haemolyticus	D	●	●	○		○	●	○	●	○	●	●	○	●	●
	T	●	●			○	●	○	●	○	○	●	○	●	●
Staphylococcus aureus (B 2198)	D	●	●	●	●	○	●	○	●	●	●	●	●	●	●
	T	●	●			○	●	○	●	●	○	●	●	●	●
Staphylococcus aureus (B 1674)	D	●	●	○		○	●	○	●	○	○	●	○	●	●
	T	●	●			○	●	○	●	●	●	●	●	●	●

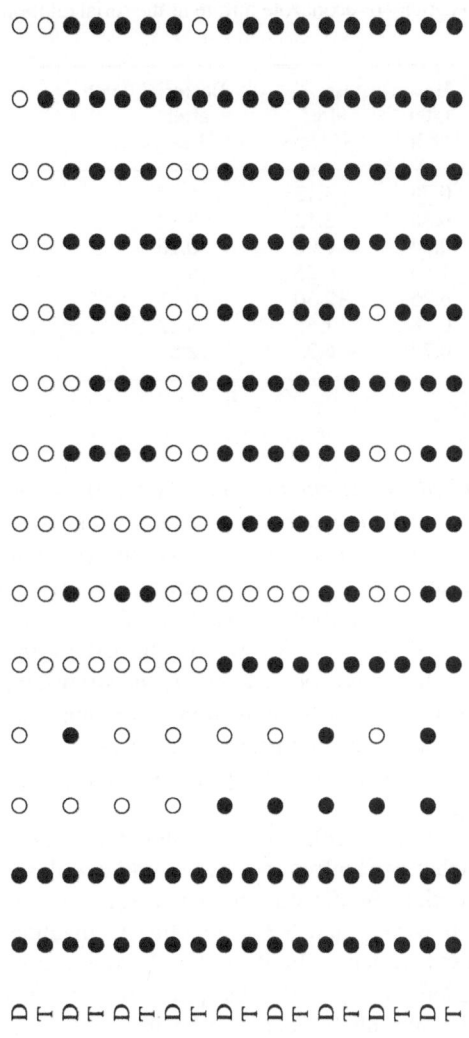

Streptococcus pyogenes	D
	T
Streptococcus faecalis	D
	T
Bacillus subtilis	D
	T
Bacillus anthracis	D
	T
Salmonella pullorum gallin	D
	T
Escherichia coli	D
	T
Pseudomonas aeruginosa	D
	T
Pasteurella pseudotuberculosis	D
	T
Bordetella bronchiseptica	D
	T

C = control, CS = control solvent (ethanol).

29

Table 7. Bacteriostatic and bactericidal activity of econazole nitrate in the serial dilution test. MIC given in μg/ml

Bacterial strain	Bacteriostasis after 48 h	after 7 Days	Bacterial death after 3 Days
Staphylococcus aureus Oxford	0.78	3.12	6.25
Staphylococcus aureus Smith	0.36	3.12	3.12
Streptococcus pyogenes A 241	0.04	0.08	0.16
Streptococcus faecalis D 5434	1.56	6.25	25
Bacillus subtilis IP – 5263	6.25	12.50	50
Bacillus anthracis IP – A 210	0.78	1.56	3.12
Actinomyces israeli (mil. Dubos)	0.78	6.25	12.5

0.78 μg/ml for two strains of *Staphylococcus aureus,* and between 0.04 and 1.56 μg/ml for *Streptococcus faecalis* and *Streptococcus pyogenes* [271, 309]. Econazole is bacteriostatic against *Actinomyces* at only 0.78 μg/ml (reading after 48 h). The bactericidal concentrations of econazole nitrate are 10–15 times higher than the bacteriostatic concentrations (see Table 7). The bactericidal and bacteriostatic activity of econazole nitrate was confirmed by the Warburg test. In *resting staphylococci* (*Staphylococcus aureus haemolyticus,* isolated from a dermatologic lesion), a significant inhibition of oxygen consumption was found starting at concentrations of 5 μg/ml. The dose-response curve obtained in these test series for econazole nitrate against *Staphylococcus aureus haemolyticus* is shown in Fig. 10.

Against proliferating staphylococci, econazole nitrate exhibited antibacterial activity only in considerably higher concentrations. At least 40 μg/ml was required to reduce oxygen consumption significantly in comparison with the controls. It must be pointed out, however, that 3.3% dimethyl formamide, which was used as a solvent in the experiment, inhibits bacterial proliferation. After introduction of the solvent alone, the proliferation phase was stopped (for details, see [242]). Against lactobacilli (Döderlein's bacilli), econazole nitrate exerted a marked inhibitory action in concentrations between 1 and 10 μg/ml. However, this is of no therapeutic relevance [284], as will be explained later (see Sect. 10.5).

3.4.3 Comparison of the Antimicrobial Activity of Econazole with Other Local Therapeutic Agents

Antimycotic Activity. During the initial phase of the evaluation of econazole, the drug was tested against positive reference substances: tolnaftate for dermatophytes, and nystatin for yeasts. The results of the comparative test series were presented in Tables 2 and 3 [309]. Econazole proved superior to tolnaftate in the control of dermatophytes, and was found to be clearly more active than nystatin against yeasts. Econazole has at least the same activity as the chemically similar miconazole [75, 271], even against the endospores of *Coccidioides immitis* [162]. Other investigators conducted comparative studies of the zones of inhibition produced by various antimycotics in cultures of *Trichophyton rubrum* [143, 144]. Either 1 or 10 µg econazole, econazole nitrate, amphotericin B, griseofulvin, nystatin, natamycin, or tolnaftate was introduced into punched holes in fungus-inoculated plates. The zones of inhibition were measured after 14 h at 23° C and an additional 48 h at 28° C. The largest inhibition zones were produced by econazole and econazole nitrate (9–12 mm or 18–20 mm in diameter, depending on the concentration). The inhibition zones for tolnaftate were 8–9 mm or 10 mm in diameter. The other substances tested had practically no effect. In a further series of tests it was determined that nystatin, undecylenic acid, hexachlorophene, zinc undecylenate, salicylic acid, and clioquinol in the same concentrations as above produced no inhibition zones in the *agar diffusion test* [220]. Griseofulvin and phenyl mercury showed inhibitory activity only at a dose of 10 µg. By contrast, clotrimazole and econazole nitrate were active in both of the concentrations tested. If the test conditions are made more difficult by seeding a mycelium into each test hole, the inhibitory effect of griseofulvin disappears. Clotrimazole and phenyl mercury produce an inhibition zone only at a dose of 10 µg. Only econazole nitrate remains active at the low dose of 1 µg.

In the *agar diffusion test with Candida albicans,* nystatin, amphotericin B, and gentian violet exhibit only slight activity (small-diameter inhibition zones), while clotrimazole and econazole are highly active [221]. Under *anaerobic* conditions on agar plates with minimal media, econazole nitrate and clotrimazole show an inhibitory effect at doses of 1, 5, and 10 µg; the extent of the effect corresponds to the action of nystatin and amphotericin B, but is superior to that of natamycin. Under *aerobic* conditions there is such a strong superficial growth of the yeasts that inhibitory effects are masked. Microscopic examination of yeasts from the boundary areas of the inhibition zones reveals the presence of damage in more than half the cells. If cells from these areas are inoculated into liquid media, no growth or reproduction is observed.

Under some conditions the activity of antimycotics not only depends on the antimicrobial activity of the drug *per se* (e. g., the minimum inhibitory concentrations for certain fungi), but is also influenced by the number of microorganisms present *(microbe-count sensitivity).* All imidazole derivatives, without exception, reveal a high microbe-count sensitivity [116]: the more microbes in the medium, the weaker the effect. The microbe-count sensitivity of the polyene antibiotics was found to be lower than that of griseofulvin, for example [233]. Comparisons of clotrimazole and miconazole with amphotericin B showed that the polyene antibiotic exhibited significantly less microbe-count sensitivity [258].

French authors [15, 16, 108] compared econazole nitrate with seven other dermatologically used antimicrobials (antimycotics) in the agar diffusion test. The tests were performed on 55 different pathogenic fungi, and the diameters of the inhibition zones were measured. As shown by the results in Table 8, econazole proved superior to all the other antimycotic agents, including the imidazole derivatives miconazole and clotrimazole which were also tested.

In assessing the results of agar diffusion tests, it must be understood that it is not just the antimicrobial activity which is being judged. The outcome of the test, i. e., the diameter of the inhibition zone, also depends on the reaction conditions, the diffusion rate of the test substance, its water solubility, and the growth rate of the test organisms [306]. Such effects are also important during the *in vivo* (therapeutic) use of the drug.

Figure 11 shows the dose-response curve for econazole nitrate, haloprogin, and chlorquinaldol applied to *Candida albicans* in the resting phase. The inhibition of oxygen consumption served as the measure of drug activity [237]. Econazole nitrate is less active than haloprogin at concentrations up to 25 μg/ml, but is superior to haloprogin at higher concentrations. After 120 min, the oxygen consumption of *Candida albicans* is practically stopped by 100 μg/ml econazole nitrate. Chlorquinaldol was found to be inferior to econazole nitrate in these test series.

Table 8. Agar diffusion tests with econazole nitrate and other antimycotics. 20 μg test substance was used in each case. The inhibition zones were measured after 48 h for the yeasts and after 7–14 days for the hyphomycetes, after [16, 108]

Species	Number of strains	Diameter of inhibition zones in mm							
		E	M	C	G	T	N	A	NA
Trichophyton rubrum	10	50–52	30–32	26–32	18–22	10–14			10–14
Epidermophyton floccosum	10	48–52	32–36	20–22	0	0			32–36
Microsporum canis	10	40–46	30–34	30–36	22–26	4–8			8–12
Trichophyton mentagrophytes	10	30–32	16–18	20–22	10–12	8–12			6–8
Candida albicans	10	20–24	18–20	12–16			22–26	8–12	12–16
Aspergillus niger	2	30–32	14–16	10–14	0	0			20–24
Madurella grisea	1	30	14	0		0			14
Phialophora pedrosoi	1	30		12		0			20
Cladosporium carrioni	1	32		6	0	0			28

E = econazole nitrate, M = miconazole nitrate, C = clotrimazole, G = griseofulvin, T = tolnaftate, N = nystatin, A = amphotericin B, NA = natamycin.

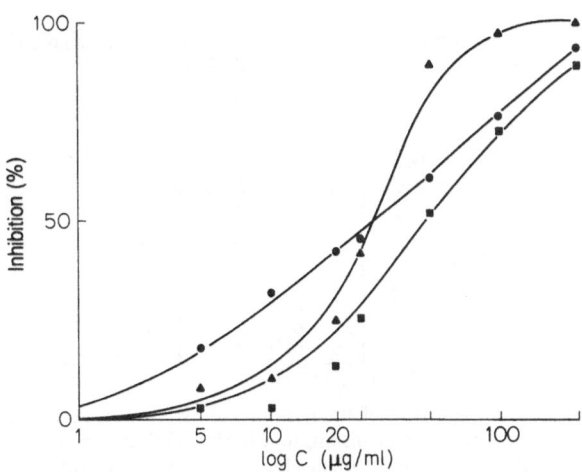

Fig. 11. Dose-response curve of econazole nitrate (▲—▲) haloprogin (●—●) and chlorquinaldol (■—■) on resting *Candida albicans*. Data in % inhibition of oxygen uptake (medium: Ringer glucose with 3.3% dimethyl formamide; test duration 120 min; absolute O_2 consumption in the controls = 184 ± 23 µl). Each flask seeded with $2 \cdot 10^6$ cells (from [237])

The Warburg test was also performed on several dermatologically important antimycotics to determine the concentrations which inhibit the oxygen consumption of resting *Candida albicans* (isolated from a dermatologic lesion) to 50% of the control value (solvent). The results are shown graphically in Fig. 12. The most active agent proved to be dodecyl-di-(β-hydroxyethyl)-benzyl-ammonium chloride, a surface-active disinfectant from the group of quaternary ammonium bases. The next most active was econazole nitrate. Higher concentrations of haloprogin and chlorquinaldol were required to achieve a 50% inhibition of oxygen consumption.

In personal investigations (unpublished) the fungicidal activities of econazole nitrate, clotrimazole, and ketoconazole were compared on a yeast strain *(Saccharomyces cerevisiae)* in the resting phase (Warburg assay, medium Ringer, pH 7.4, with glucose and 3.3% dimethyl formamide, oxygen consumption over 90 min periods: 130 µl). Econazole nitrate inhibited oxygen consumption by 92%, clotrimazole by 60% and ketoconazole by 10%; all imidazoles were tested in a concentration of 100 µg/ml. The marked superiority of econazole nitrate over ketoconazole was confirmed in a further test series on *Candida albicans:* in media with Ringer-glucose, ketoconazole exhibits only about half the activity of econazole nitrate; however, this superiority markedly diminished when serum was added to the medium (personal experiments by Warburg assay, measurement of oxygen consumption of resting yeasts; unpublished). In similar experimental studies in vitro, econazole nitrate was compared to N-148/76 (formula given in Fig. 8). On resting *Candida albicans* (oxygen consumption 163 µl/90 min), econazole nitrate inhibited respiration by 34%,

33

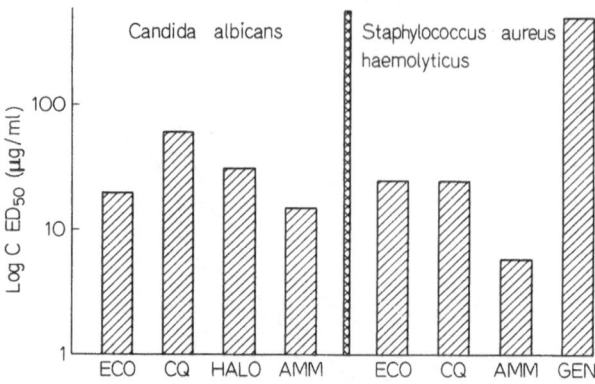

Fig. 12. Comparison of the concentrations of various antimicrobials that cause a 50% inhibition of oxygen consumption in the Warburg test on resting organisms. (Test duration 90 min; medium: Ringer glucose with 3.3% diemthyl formamide; control values for *Candida albicans* 184 ± 23 μl O$_2$/90 min, for *Staphylococcus aureus haemolyticus* 111 ± 12 μl O$_2$/120 min) (from [237]). AMM = dodecyl-di-(β-hydroxyethyl)-benzylammonium chloride, GEN = gentamicin, CQ = chlorquinaldol, HALO = haloprogin, ECO = econazole nitrate

whereas N-148/76 acted much weaker and provoked an inhibition by 10% only; both substances were assayed in concentrations of 30 μg/ml (personal investigations, unpublished).

The comparative investigations discussed here would indicate that econazole is among the most active of the antimycotic agents. The better showing of econazole nitrate in the diffusion tests is not necessarily due to a stronger antimicrobial activity *per se* in comparison with the structurally similar substances miconazole and clotrimazole. More favorable physical properties surely contribute to the better test results. But physical factors (rapid diffusion, good solubility) are also important during therapeutic use. From this standpoint, the results of the agar diffusion tests are of considerable practical relevance.

Antibacterial Activity. In the initial series of tests of the antimicrobial properties of econazole, a comparison with benzyl penicillin showed that the two agents have approximately equal bactericidal and bacteriostatic activities against gram-positive bacteria (Table 6). Penicillin is effective to some degree against gram-negative bacteria, while econazole is inactive against these organisms. The inhibition values of econazole against staphylococci and streptococci are lower than those of clotrimazole [216, 309]. In the agar diffusion test, econazole nitrate produces larger zones of inhibition in staphylococci than clotrimazole, and even somewhat larger zones than miconazole nitrate [14]. In interpreting these results of the agar plate diffusion test, the same considerations apply as were discussed on p. 32.

It is a rather difficult task to give a relevant judgement on an antifungal substance by considering the minimum inhibitory concentrations in vitro. Data

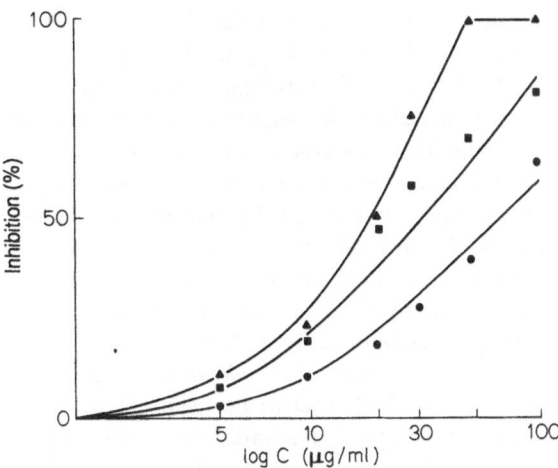

Fig. 13. Dose-response curve of econazole nitrate (▲—▲), haloprogin (●—●) and chlorquinaldol (■—■) on resting staphylococci *(Staphylococcus aureus haemolyticus)*. Data in % inhibition of oxygen uptake relative to the controls (medium: Ringer glucose with 3.3% dimethyl formamide; test duration 120 min; oxygen consumption in the controls = 111 ± 12 μl). Each flask seeded with 10^7 cells (from [237])

from different groups of investigators never can be compared directly. In the case of econazole nitrate, for example, minimum inhibitory concentrations against dermatophytes vary between 0.001 and 100 μg/ml! The respective values for *Candida albicans* reported in the literature range between 0.6 and 10 μg/ml. The results of experiments designed to determine the minimum inhibitory concentrations *in vitro* depend upon the growth medium and upon the size of the inoculum, just to mention the two most important factors. One may conclude that the minimum inhibitory concentrations are indicative of the relative antifungal activities of different substances *in vitro*, when assayed in the *same* series. The main point of an evaluation, however, will always be the therapeutic assay.

Figure 13 shows the dose-response curves for the action of econazole nitrate, haloprogin, and chlorquinaldol on the oxygen consumption of *Staphylococcus aureus haemolyticus*. The decrease in oxygen consumption relative to the control (solvent) served as the measure of antibacterial activity. Concentrations from 1 to 100 μg/ml were tested. In the range from 5 to 100 μg/ml, econazole proved more effective than the other two antimicrobials. Up to a concentration of 25 μg/ml, the activity of chlorquinaldol was only slightly below that of econazole nitrate. Haloprogin exhibited a much lower antibacterial activity than econazole nitrate and chlorquinaldol. The dose-response curves in Fig. 13 pertain to a time period of 120 min. It should also be noted that the onset of action of econazole nitrate occurred within 15 min after the start of the test. In the case of haloprogin, antibacterial action was first evident after

30 min. Chlorquinaldol was also slower than econazole nitrate in initiating its inhibitory action on the oxygen consumption of the staphylococci.

The Warburg test was again employed to determine the concentration of some dermatologically important antibacterial agents which would cause a 50% inhibition of oxygen consumption relative to the control (solvent). As with *Candida albicans* (see p. 34), the quaternary ammonium base showed the greatest activity (Fig. 12). Econazole nitrate and chlorquinaldol were about equally effective (about 25 µg/ml required to produce 50% inhibition). The necessary concentrations of haloprogin were almost four times higher. Still higher concentrations of antibiotics were needed: 500 µg/ml gentamicin and 2000 µg/ml sodium fusidate. Neomycin exhibited no inhibitory effect on the oxygen consumption of *Staphylococcus aureus haemolyticus* in the resting phase, but was highly active against proliferating staphylococci even in concentrations of 0.5 µg/ml. The problems of demonstrating the effects of econazole on proliferating bacteria were discussed in Sect. 3.4.3. Thus, it cannot be compared with neomycin in the Warburg test.

On a pathogenetic strain of *Staphylococcus aureus haemolyticus,* a comparison was made by manometric technique between ketoconazole, econazole, and clotrimazole; the concentration of each substance was 50 µg/ml (personal experimental series, unpublished). Econazole and clotrimazole inhibited oxygen consumption of the staphylococci to about the same degree (41% and 45%, respectively), whereas ketoconazole was significantly less effective (inhibition by 16% only). The advantage of ketoconazole must be seen in its absorption upon oral use.

The same technique was used to compare econazole nitrate with another imidazole derivative, N-148/76 (formula in Fig. 8), The concentrations were 40 µg/ml. Oxygen consumption of the resting staphylococci amounted to 110 µl/90 min in the controls. Econazole nitrate exerted an inhibitory action of 46%, whereas N-148/76 inhibited oxygen consumption by 25%, only (personal experiments, unpublished).

According to the results of the tests described, econazole has good activity against gram-positive bacteria. The antibacterial action of econazole nitrate is slightly stronger than that of miconazole nitrate and even stronger than that of clotrimazole, at least as regards the results of agar diffusion tests [16, 108]. This would also indicate a stronger antibacterial action during clinical use. 1% isoconazole nitrate – as active against bacteria as isoconazole – has been reported to be more effective against bacteria on human skin than 1% clotrimazole [355].

The results of the Warburg test demonstrate that econazole nitrate is at least equal to the other dermatologically used broad-spectrum antimicrobials in its antibacterial action, as far as gram-positive organisms are concerned. But since it is the gram-positive bacteria which cause secondary infections in inflamed skin lesions and especially in superficial dermatophytoses (tinea) and candidoses, the activity of the imidazoles against gram-positive bacteria greatly enhances their value in the treatment of mycotic infections (see Sect. 9).

3.4.4 Activity Against Protozoa (Trichomonads)

All antitrichomonal drugs available for systemic use (metronidazole, tinidazole, see Table 1 and Fig. 3) are derived from the family of imidazole derivatives. It was natural, therefore, to test clotrimazole, miconazole, and econazole for their antitrichomonal activity as well. Especially in the treatment of vaginitis (colpitis), a concurrent activity against *Candida albicans* or other yeasts and trichomonads *(Trichomonas vaginalis)* is of great importance.

The minimum inhibitory concentrations of econazole nitrate for *Trichomonas vaginalis* are between four and ten times those of metronidazole, the positive trichomonacidal reference substance.

Econazole has not been directly compared with the trichomonacidal concentrations or polyene antibiotics, which, unlike metronidazole, can be applied only locally. The inhibitory concentrations of the polyene antibiotics against trichomonads range from 0.1 µg/ml for hamycin to 40 µg/ml for natamycin (the duration of exposure must be taken into account, of course).

When econazole is administered systemically, trichomonacidal concentrations cannot be produced in the tissues. When applied locally, however, it has proved effective in preventing on overgrowth of trichomonads.

The clinical success rate of clotrimazole and miconazole in the treatment of trichomonal infections is from 50% to 75%, with a duration of treatment of only 1 week in most cases. Recent infections respond better than long-standing ones [30, 156, 277]. No controlled clinical studies are yet available on the use of econazole in the treatment of trichomonal infections. It is assumed that the success rate would correspond roughly to that of clotrimazole (50% cure rate, [156, 277]) and miconazole (12 cures among 16 female patients [30]).

4 General Microbiology of Imidazole Derivatives for Local Application

4.1 Preliminary Remarks

Clotrimazole, miconazole, and econazole exhibit a broad spectrum of antimycotic activity and inhibit the growth of dermatophytes, yeasts, and molds. They are thus suited for the treatment of all mycoses (mycotic infections) of the skin and mucous membranes (broad-spectrum antimycotics).

Clotrimazole, miconazole, and econazole have also demonstrated a clinically relevant activity against gram-positive bacteria, which justifies their inclusion in the group of broad-spectrum antimicrobials. Because gram-positive bacteria play a major role on body surfaces and are important as concomitant pathogens or secondarily infecting organisms in mycotic infections (dermatophytoses [149] and candidoses [195], the imidazole derivatives are particularly well suited for the treatment of mycoses.

No *qualitative* difference in antimicrobial spectrum can be found between clotrimazole, miconazole, and econazole [309, 313]; the *quantitative* differences were discussed in Sect. 3.4.3. The mechanism of the antimicrobial action of the three compounds is assumed to be the same.

The broad spectrum of clotrimazole, miconazole, and econazole suggests that there is no *specific* interaction with the structural components or metabolic pathways of microbes. But a more nonspecific, generally "cytotoxic" mode of action could – in theory – also damage animal cells (i. e., the host organism during infections); this is much less likely in the case of "specific" antibiotic actions. It is for this reason that the good tolerance of the imidazole derivatives was surprising.

4.2 Mode of Action

4.2.1 Morphological Findings

The imidazole derivatives clotrimazole, miconazole, and econazole act by damaging the membranes of bacterial and fungal cells (Figs. 7 and 8); both the cellular and subcellular membranes are affected.

38

After *13-h exposure* to econazole (0.05 μg/ml = 1.1 · 10^{-7} mol/liter), the cell wall of *Trichophyton rubrum* exhibits a diminished electron density. The mitochondria also show structural changes: They lose their rod shape and become more spherical; the mitochondrial cristae exhibit vesicular structures and finally undergo lytic decomposition. This finding can be explained by assuming the dissolution of all internal membranes of the mitochondria. After another 13 h, the nuclear structures become poorly defined. They can no longer be differentiated into chromatin, matrix, and nucleolus.

Twenty-six hours' exposure to econazole at a concentration of 0.1 μg/ml (= 2.2 · 10^{-7} mol/liter) causes irreversible damage to the organelles of the *Trichophyton rubrum* cell: decomposition of the ribosomes and mitochondria, disintegration of the nuclei, and detachment of the plasmalemma from the cell wall. Vesicles appear in the region of the cell wall and in the space between the cell wall and plasma membrane.

The higher the concentration of econazole, the more rapidly these changes develop. One peculiarity is the finding of an increased electron density in the cell wall after exposure to econazole at a concentration between 25 and 75 μg/ml. It is assumed that such high concentrations lead to an outward diffusion of osmiophilic decomposition products from subcellular membranous structures. These osmiophilic substances (lipids) are then deposited in the cell wall (cf. photomicrographs in Figs. 14 and 15).

The observed changes suggest the following mechanism of action of econazole on dermatophytes:
1) Econazole increases the permeability of the fungal cell.
2) Econazole enters the cytoplasm.
3) Econazole damages all membranous structures in the cytoplasm.
4) The resulting degeneration (decomposition) products are either isolated in the form of vesicles or accumulate in extracellular regions.
5) Lipid substances diffuse outward and are deposited in the cell wall [220].

The morphological changes produced in yeasts by econazole and other imidazole derivatives are similar to those produced in mycelial fungi. For example, exposing *Candida albicans* to miconazole [63] or clotrimazole [139, 140] leads to a segregation of cytoplasmic components; this was interpreted as a sign of detoxification or the result of increased plasmalemma synthesis following injury. Low concentrations cause mainly a proliferation of structures at the cell periphery, an increase in the number of peroxisomes, and an increase in the cell volume [64, 316]. These changes must be interpreted either as a sign of a permeability disturbance [140, 288, 316] or as the result of adaptation by the yeast cell to a depression of its metabolism. The latter hypothesis is supported by the observation of accumulated membrane particles between the cell wall and plasmalemma and by the retention of substances in the cytoplasm. But perhaps the proliferation in the membrane region should be interpreted as only a partial symptom of a nonspecific defense reaction.

After 12 h exposure to 10 μg econazole/ml (= 2.2 · 10^{-5} mol/liter), 50-nm vacuoles appear in the cytoplasm of *Candida albicans,* caused by the dissolution

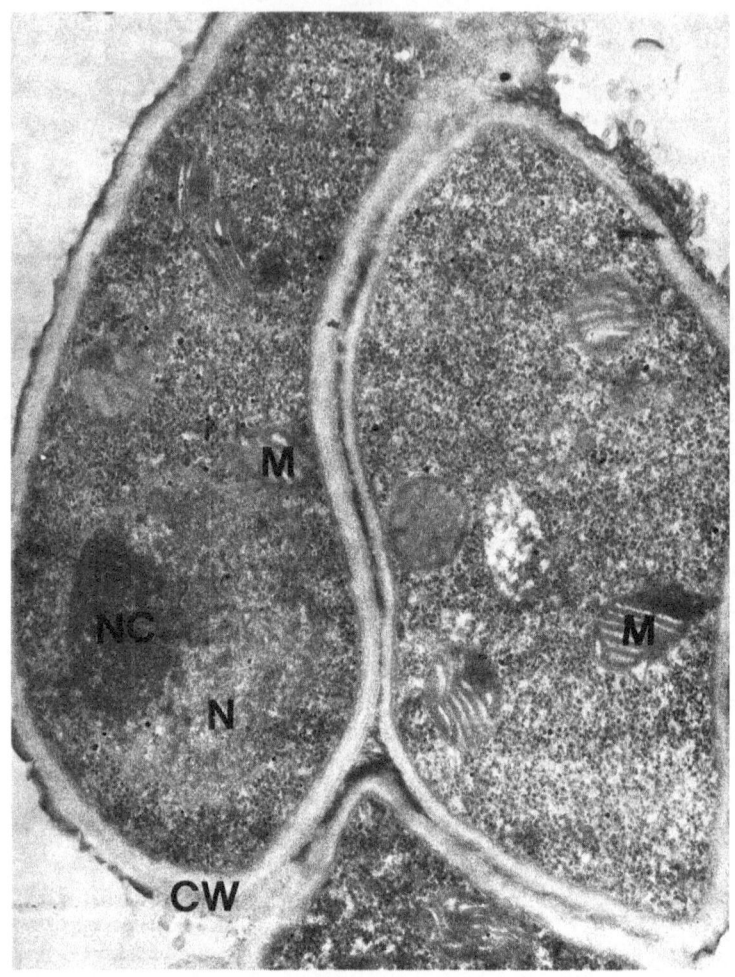

Fig. 14. *Trichophyton rubrum.* Ultrathin section through untreated cells. N = nucleus, NC = nucleolus, CW = cell wall, M = mitochondria (x 26,000)

of normal constituents. The cell walls show density variations which can be detected only by special techniques [223]. Also the plasmalemma is severely damaged [225]. The changes, or the destruction of the mitochondria and the accumulation of lipids, resemble the disturbances caused by econazole in dermatophytes (Figs. 16–19).

Thus, econazole leads to a disturbance of cell permeability and intraplasmatic membrane changes in yeasts as well in dermatophytes. This has the effect of blocking RNA, protein, and lipid metabolism [221].

When applied therapeutically (in man or animals), the imidazole derivatives produce changes in the infecting fungi which are similar to the changes

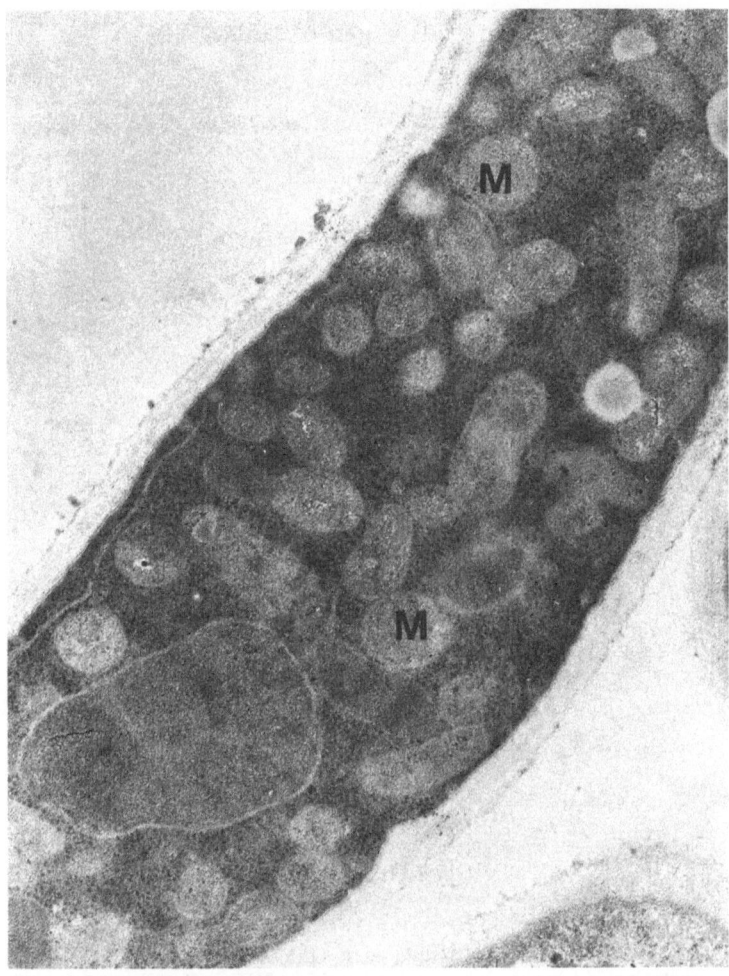

Fig. 15. *Trichophyton rubrum.* After 26-h exposure to econazole in a concentration of 0.05µg/ml, the number and volume of the mitochondria (M) are considerably increased. Most of the cristae are lysed (x 27,000)

observed *in vitro* [323, 324]. Findings are already available on morphological changes in molds: In mice with renal aspergillosis (infected with *Aspergillus fumigatus*), the fungal cell membrane shows an undulating contour after the start of systemic clotrimazole therapy; electron-dense and osmiophilic structures appear in the cell wall, and nuclear changes are evident [323]. This corresponds in large measure to the changes observed in *Trichophyton rubrum* and *Candida albicans* treated with econazole *in vitro.* The introduction of econazole nitrate into an infected vagina provoked the "typical" morphological changes in *Candida albicans* and in gram-positive bacteria [222, 224, 354].

41

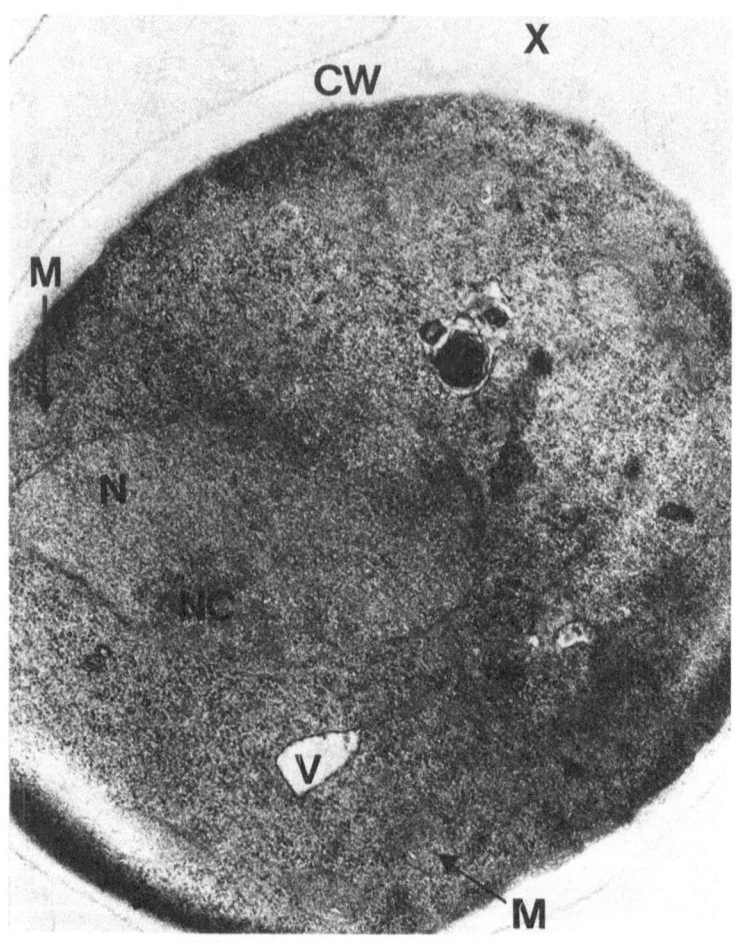

Fig. 16. *Candida albicans.* Ultrathin section through an untreated cell. N = nucleus, NC = nucleolus, V = vacuole, M = mitochondria. CW = cell wall with "scar" (X) following blastospore formation (x 25,000)

4.2.2 Biochemical Effects

Even the initial studies on the biochemical changes produced in fungi by the action of imidazole derivatives revealed a massive disturbance of cell membrane permeability, with the leakage of potassium ions, sodium ions, and low-molecular phosphates from the cell. The final dissolution of the cell is preceded by a protein loss [139, 140, 315, 343]. Enzymes are also lost from the cell a few minutes after the start of exposure to econazole [343]. Based on the massive disturbance of *transport mechanisms* observed, it was hypothesized that clotrimazole, miconazole, and econazole bind to unsaturated fatty acids of the

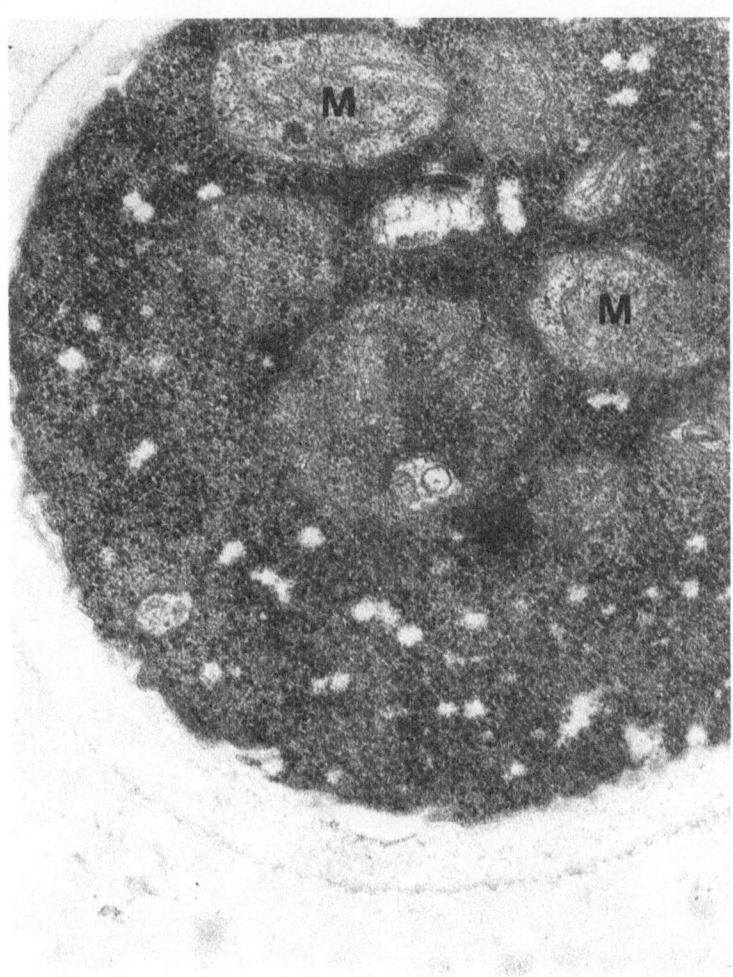

Fig. 17. *Candida albicans.* Twelve-hour exposure to econazole (10 µg/ml) led to an increase in the number and volume of the mitochondria (M). Lytic processes produce localized electron-transparent regions in the cytoplasm (x 43,000)

lecithin molecules in the cytoplasmic membrane [338]. A reaction with phospholipids could satisfactorily account for such a massive disruption of transport mechanisms.

Studies on the behavior of various important *enzyme activities* of fungal cells treated with imidazole derivatives led to the development of the *peroxide poisoning hypothesis:* Imidazole derivatives inhibit cytochrome-*C* peroxidase and activate catalase in fungistatically active concentrations. Fungicidal concentrations cause the complete inhibition of cytochrome-*C* peroxidase and catalase. However, NADH oxidase still exhibits a high activity, and peroxides

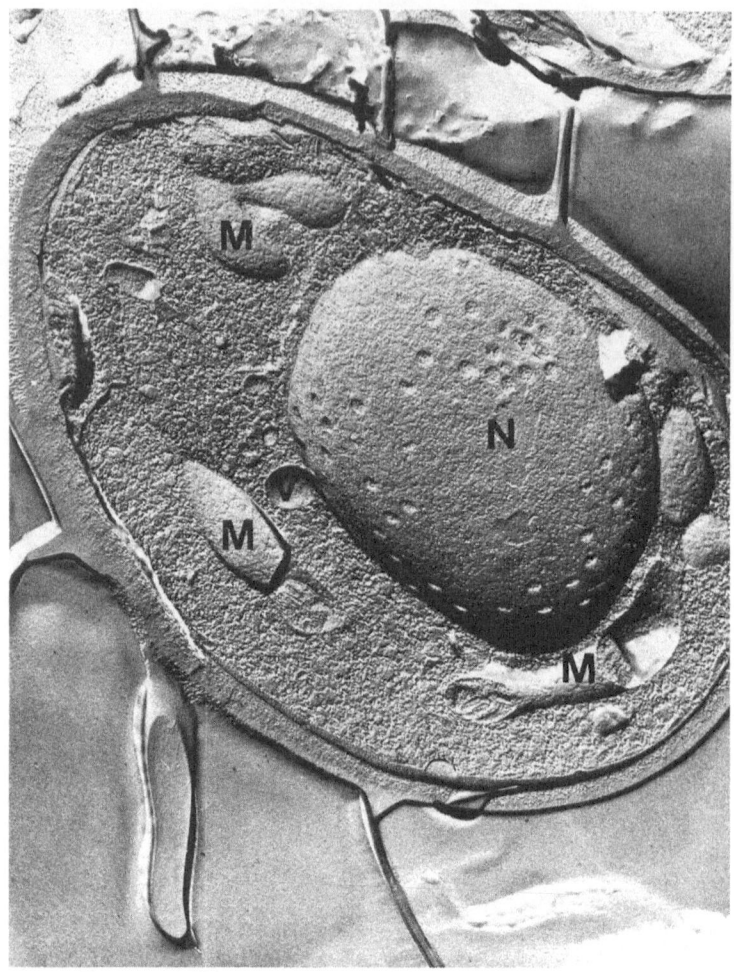

Fig. 18. Freeze-fractured *Candida albicans* cell (untreated, unfixed). The fracture across the protoplasts shows the ribosome-rich and therefore coarse-grained cytoplasm containing mitochondria (M), vacuoles (V), and the nucleus (N), whose membrane is studded with nuclear pores (x 17,500)

continue to be produced. These peroxides may be responsible for the massive damage which finally leads to cell death [63]. Personal investigations revealed an inhibtory action of econazole nitrate on glucose-6-phosphate dehydrogenase activity (EC 1.1.1.49); various phosphatases, peptidases, and β-glucuronidase remained uninfluenced [243].

Recent investigations demonstrated an interference of the imidazole antifungals with ergosterol formation *in vivo* and *in vitro* [112, 317]; these data were mainly collected in *Candida albicans*. The conversion of 24-methylenedi-

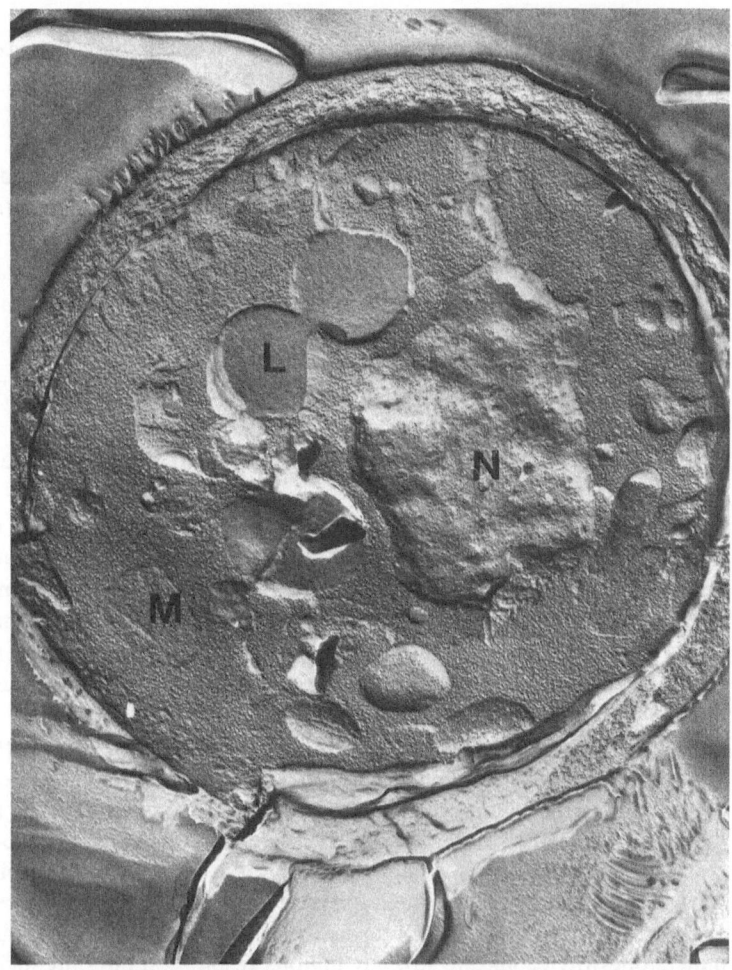

Fig. 19. Freeze-fractured *Candida albicans* cell after 24-h exposure to econazole (10 µg/ ml). The ribosomes are dissolved, giving the cytoplasm a fine-grained structure. Disturbances of cell metabolism cause lipid deposits (L). The nucleus (N) and the interior of the mitochondria (M) are largely destroyed (x 17,500)

hydrolanosterol to ergosterol seems to be blocked in the presence of imidazole derivatives; which step of the removal of the 14-α methyl group from lanosterol is attacked needs to be elucidated. As ergosterol is the most important sterol for most fungi, it may be assumed that an accumulation of sterols with a substitute on the carbon atom at position 14 provokes permeability changes (damage in various membrane systems). In the case of ketoconazole, an inhibition of cholesterol biosynthesis is effectuated in animals, too; however, this effect occurs only when high doses are administered. It should be recalled that fungal cells rely much more on their own ergosterol synthesis than mammalian cells which can use sterols from the surrounding medium.

In very low concentrations that are still growth-inhibiting, econazole interferes with the incorporation of adenine, guanine, and hypoxanthine into macromolecules, which is in good agreement with the first hypothesis regarding the action of benzimidazole (see Sect. 2.5.1). In low concentration (0.01 µg/ml, or $2 \cdot 10^{-8}$ mol/liter), econazole does not interfere with the uptake of glucose, leucine and glycine by *Candida albicans*. The action of econazole (and other imidazoles) must be distinguished from that of actinomycin D with respect to the disturbance of purine incorporation: actinomycin D inhibits only the *incorporation* of purines into ribonucleic acids without disturbing their intracellular *uptake*. Econazole inhibits the passage of purines through the cell membrane.

Econazole interferes with the permeation of yeast cells in both directions. This could be shown for the enzyme maltase (exit from the cell) and for a chromogenic substrate for intracellular maltase activity (entry of the substrate into the cell with a resulting coloration of the cell) [343].

Econazole leads to a strong inhibition of respiration [143, 144, 145, 241], but to only a slight impairment of glycolysis. For example, econazole (50 µg/ml) provoked in one series of tests a complete cessation of respiration, but lony a 25% inhibition of glycolysis (fermentation). Lower concentrations (10 or 20 µg/ml) had a smaller effect on respiration, but augmented glycolysis. This was interpreted as a decoupling of oxidative phosphorylation. Interestingly, this effect cannot be produced by miconazole [143].

The respiration of yeast cells, like all cell respiration, is based on the actions of respiratory-chain enzymes. These enzymes are packed closely together in the mitochondrial inner membrane. Disturbances of this membrane lead to an inhibition of respiration. Econazole and miconazole cause damage to the mitochondrial inner membrane; clotrimazole reportedly lacks this ability [143, 144]. The enzymes of glycolysis differ from the enzymes of the respiratory chain in that they are not bound to membranous structures. It can now be understood why econazole strongly inhibits respiration but only slightly influences glycolysis. The slight inhibition of glycolysis is probably based on a loss of important metabolites from the cell.

The inhibition of respiration by econazole was found to be pH-dependent. The greatest activty was observed at pH 6.85, an almost neutral pH. Shifts of the pH value in an acidic or alkaline direction required higher concentrations of econazole to achieve the same antimicrobial effect. At pH 4.35, for example, a ten times higher concentration is needed [143, 144]. The decrease in the activity of econazole in a strongly basic medium is probably due to its poorer solubility. The loss of activity in an acidic environment is due to a protonation of the imidazole core [144]. The fungitoxicity of imidazole dervatives depends mainly on the substituents at the imino nitrogen. They are most active fungicidally when the substituted atom possesses a tetrahedral structure, thereby creating an electron affinity. In an acidic medium, on the other hand, proton attachment occurs; this reduces the antimicrobial activity of the compound.

In morphological studies (see above), it has been demonstrated that imidazole antifungals damage mitochondrial membranes. This could be confirmed in biochemical studies [245]. Exposure of rat liver mitochondria to econazole nitrate (50 μg/ml for maximal effect) leads to a liberation of mitochondrial enzymes into the supernatant, indicating that damage of the mitochondrial membranes has taken place.

4.2.3 Sites of Action in the Cell

According to the results of the previously mentioned investigations, clotrimazole, miconazole, and econazole act on the structural components of important membranous systems within the fungal cell, most probably on the unsaturated fatty acid acyl moiety of the membrane phospholipids [338, 339] Imidazole derivatives cause damage to the plasma membrane as well as to subcellular membranes. The resulting changes lead to the death of the cell.

Unlike the polyene antibiotics, the imidazole derivatives do not act on sterol bodies in the cell wall (ergosterol, cholesterol), although they inhibit ergosterol synthesis. Besides, the cell walls of bacteria (gram-positive cocci) are devoid of ergosterol and cholesterol, and so such constituents are not available to react with the imidazoles.

The primary factor to be considered is a reaction between the imidazole derivatives and the phospholipids. The exact nature of this reaction has not yet been established.

4.3 Resistance and Tolerance

Many antimicrobial agents which were extremely effective when introduced into medical therapy have become less and less effective with duration of use. The classic example of this is the use of penicillin in the treatment of gonorrhea: Initially, a single injection of 150000 units was sufficient to cure the infection. Today, ever-increasing doses must be administered, for the susceptibility of gonococci to penicillin is continuously declining. There are now β-lactamase-forming strains of gonococci which are completely resistant to penicillin. Such strains have already been detected in 12 countries. It is only a matter of time before penicillin is completely ineffective in the treatment of gonorrhea.

The situation is not quite so blatant in the case of skin-surface microorganisms. But here, too, the resistance quotas are so high, especially in hospitals ("hospitalism"), that local antibiotic therapy is practiced less often. Due to uncertainty over the concentrations which actually take effect, local treatment is considered highly favorable for the development of resistance. Particularly questionable is the practice of diluting ointments and creams which contain both a glucocorticoid (whose dilution matters little) as well as an antibiotic.

The declining clinical efficacy of an antimicrobial agent can be verified *in vitro:* the minimum inhibitory concentrations increase, based on tests in large populations, and "resistant" mutants develop. Such a phenomenon may be due either to *resistance* or to *tolerance*. The culturing of microbes in nutrient media with gradually increasing concentrations of the antimicrobial agent leads to the development of organisms with increased resistance to the drug. Subthreshold doses during clinical usage have the same effect.

The nomenclature of resistance and tolerance is not entirely uniform. In general, the term *primary resistance* is used when a certain group of microbes out of an otherwise susceptible strain responds to the antimicrobial agent only at relatively high concentrations or, if resistance is total, does not respond at all — this without any prior contact with the drug. *Resistance* alone refers to diminished susceptibility as a result of one or more prior contacts with the drug. Resistant strains can be cultured *in vitro* by subjecting them to numerous passages over nutrient media with increasing amounts of the antimicrobial drug. Resistance is genetically fixed. *Tolerance* is different from resistance. "Tolerant" organisms also develop when cultured in media containing the drug. But if the organisms are transferred to media that are free of the drug, their original high sensitivity to the drug returns after a few passages. In this case the resistance was not genetically fixed. Due to the growing importance of the resistance problem in medicine, studies are done as soon as a new class of antimicrobials is introduced to determine whether resistance or tolerance will be likely to occur.

So far in the laboratory, it has been inpossible to culture dermatophytes *(Trichophyton rubrum)* or yeasts *(Candida albicans)* which are resistant to econazole or clotrimazole, even when as many as 22 passages were employed. A tolerance could be induced in *Torulopsis glabrata,* but the fungus could not be made resistant to the drugs [143, 144, 344]. The same statement applies to *Candida albicans.* According to previous *clinical* reports, not a single case of primary resistance to any of the imidazole derivatives has yet been documented. However, in *one* patient, after prolonged systemic administration of miconazole, a resistant strain of *Candida albicans* was observed [129]; the resistance was parallel to miconazole and econazole.

It can thus be assumed that no resistance or tolerance problems are associated at present with the use of econazole, miconazole, or clotrimazole. Numerous test results justify the hope that these agents will maintain their high effectiveness in the future. Furthermore, an adaptation to toxic actions which alter important surface structures is more difficult to conceive than adjustments of the metabolism in response to antibiotic actions.

4.4 Interactions with Other Compounds

4.4.1 Preliminary Remarks

Drugs are not used in pure form in local therapy, but are incorporated into various vehicles (ointments, creams, powders, tinctures, lotions). It is important to determine whether reactions take place between the drug and the vehicle. Such reactions could significantly impair the clinical efficacy of the preparation. Corresponding tests are an important part of bioavailability studies.

Another type of interaction must be considered when the preparation is applied to the outer skin: interactions with substances on the skin surface (proteins, lipids). The main proteins to be considered are keratin and the serum proteins found on the skin surface in severe inflammation. The principal lipids are those secreted by the sebaceous glands. The possible interactions between imidazole derivatives and lipids merit special consideration, for these drugs are capable of reacting with the lipids of cellular and subcellular membranes (see Sect. 4.2). The final question to be asked is whether imidazole antifungals can be applied locally together with other substances. This must also be tested first *in vitro*.

4.4.2 Proteins

Most investigators were unable to detect any significant decrease in the antimicrobial activity of econazole in the presence of serum [143, 309]. Only one research group found an increase in the minimum inhibitory concentrations of econazole (base) for *Candida albicans* and gram-positive cocci in the presence of 10% bovine serum [271].

Clotrimazole and miconazole have also shown diminished activity in the presence of serum in only a few studies. Most investigators report an absence of protein sensitivity. Thus, one may assume that the antimycotic activity of externally applied imidazole derivatives is not significantly reduced when used on weeping skin lesions.

4.4.3 Lipids

The surface of the skin is covered by a thin lipid film. These lipids originate mostly from the sebaceous glands and to a lesser extent from cellular differentiation processes. At the excretory ducts of the sebaceous glands (follicular openings) are small pools of oil whose contents become spread over the skin surface by the friction of clothing or the hands.

Lipids could inhibit the action of econazole by coating the fungal cell wall with a lipid film which protects against the action of econazole, or by reacting directly with econazole to form antimicrobially inactive products.

49

The cell wall of microbes is composed of polysaccharides and lipids; the accumulation of further lipids is entirely conceivable. The action of econazole apparently stems in part from a reaction with lipids in the plasma membrane. If the same lipids are present in the reaction medium, inactivation could result.

When tests are conducted to determine whether skin-surface lipids can inhibit the action of econazole, it is necessary first to calculate the quantities involved in the reaction. A maximum of 0.3 mg lipid substances is present on 1 cm^2 human skin [300]. This 0.3 mg is composed of 0.012 mg cholesterol and cholesterol esters (4%), 0.0180 mg triglycerides (60%), and 0.108 mg waxes and squalene (36%).

External preparations are applied in a thin layer and are partially rubbed in. Under the least favorable conditions, it can be assumed that a 0.1-mm-thick layer of the preparation actually comes in contact with the skin surface. A 0.1-mm-thick layer corresponds to a quantity of 0.01 cm^3 ointment or cream per square centimeter, which in 1% preparations (clotrimazole, econazole nitrate) contains 0.1 mg of the drug.

It must thus be assumed that under clinical conditions, 0.1 mg econazole nitrate will react with 0.3 mg lipid mixture/cm^2 skin surface. Accordingly, the action of econazole must be tested in the presence of a lipid concentration that is three times higher.

The Warburg test was performed on resting *Saccharomyces cerevisiae* and *Candida albicans* to determine whether the action of econazole nitrate is antagonized by the presence of a "synthetic" sebum (mixture of cholesterol, triglycerides, and squalene in a ratio of $1:15:19$) in a three fold concentration. Econazole nitrate was used at a concentration of 40 µg/ml, and the lipid mixture at 120 µg lipids/ml. No decrease in the activity of econazole was observed. The same observation was made in tests with natural sebum. Further tests were done with the same organisms to determine whether *higher* concentrations of lipids could inhibit the action of econazole. It was found that cholesterol as well as triglycerides and squalene could significantly reduce the activity of econazole nitrate (40 µg/ml) in concentrations of 200 and 400 µg/ml. The results of the tests are shown graphically in Fig. 20. They indicate that the antimicrobial activity of econazole will not be hampered by skin-surface lipids during the course of external dermatologic therapy.

4.4.4 Glucocorticoids

On the basis of clinical considerations (see Sect. 13), the combined use of antimicrobial agents and glucocorticoids seems quite favorable. Before such combinations are used, however, it must be certain that no antagonistic interactions will occur. Such interactions between an antimicrobial agent and a glucocorticoid could occur by various mechanisms:
1) Direct chemical reaction (precipitation, formation of complexes)
2) Mutual acceleration of inactivation

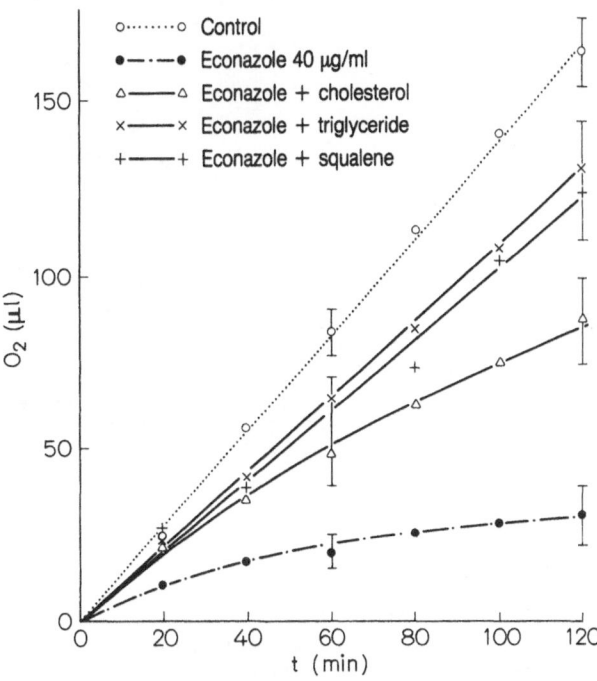

Fig. 20. Oxygen consumption of resting *Saccharomyces cerevisiae* under the influence of econazole nitrate with and without a tenfold concentration of cholesterol, triglycerides, or squalene. Medium: Ringer with 3.3% dimethyl formamide. Substrate: glucose. Lipid concentrations: 400 µg/ml

3) Physicochemical interaction (competitive inhibiton, receptor blockage, formation of protective film)
4) Biologic antagonism (glucocorticoids in low concentrations stimulate microbe metabolism [235])
5) Mutual inhibition of permeation

Only a few studies have been done to date on the interactions between imidazole derivatives and glucocorticoids. This may be due in part to technical difficulties (use of two substances that are difficult to dissolve).

A serial dilution test was performed to study the antimicrobial activity of isoconazole in the presence of various concentrations of diflucortolone valerianate [146]. The presence of difluorocortolone valerianate in one-tenth the concentration of isoconazole did not reduce its antimicrobial activity against *Staphylococcus aureus*, *Candida albicans*, and *Trichophyton mentagrophytes*. Higher concentrations of difluorocortolone valerianate reduced the antimicrobial activity of isoconazole: studies done by the "chessboard" technique showed that a four times higher concentration of the steroid is needed to reduce the antibacterial effect of isoconazole against *Staphylococcus aureus*, and at least a 50 times higher concentration to reduce its effect against *Tricho-*

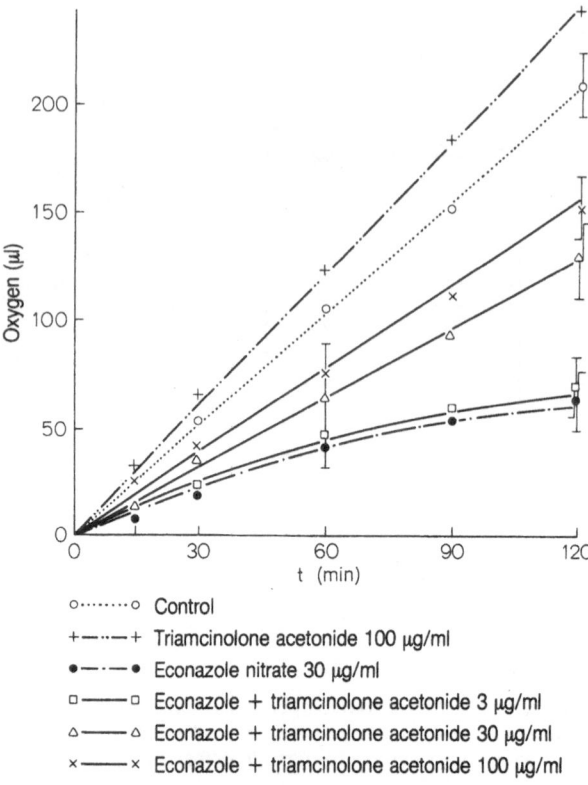

○┈┈┈┈○ Control
+—··—+ Triamcinolone acetonide 100 μg/ml
●—·—● Econazole nitrate 30 μg/ml
□————□ Econazole + triamcinolone acetonide 3 μg/ml
△————△ Econazole + triamcinolone acetonide 30 μg/ml
×————× Econazole + triamcinolone acetonide 100 μg/ml

Fig. 21. Oxygen consumption of resting *Saccharomyces cerevisiae* under the influence of econazole nitrate and triamcinolone acetonide in various concentrations. Medium: Ringer glucose with 3.3% dimethyl formamide

phyton mentagrophytes. The antimicrobial activity of clotrimazole is not impaired by the presence of dexamethasone [217].

Some investigations dealt with the action of econazole nitrate, isoconazole nitrate, and chlormidazole on *Saccharomyces cerevisiae, Candida albicans,* and *Staphylococcus aureus haemolyticus* in the presence of hydrocortisone, fluocinolone acetonide, or triamcinolone acetonide. In the case of *Saccharomyces cerevisiae,* the action of econazole was significantly inhibited as soon as hydrocortisone or triamcinolone acetonide was applied in at least the concentration of the econazole nitrate (Fig. 21). This effect was observed for *Candida albicans* only when the steroid concentration was at least ten times higher (Fig. 22). However, a doubly fluorinated glucocorticoid (difluorocortolone valerianate) slightly weakened the effect of econazole and isoconazole on *Candida albicans* when used in the *same* concentration. Fluocinolone acetonide reduced the effect of chlormidazole on *Candida albicans* only very slightly [249]. Neither hydrocortisone nor singly or doubly fluorinated glucocorticoids could alter the

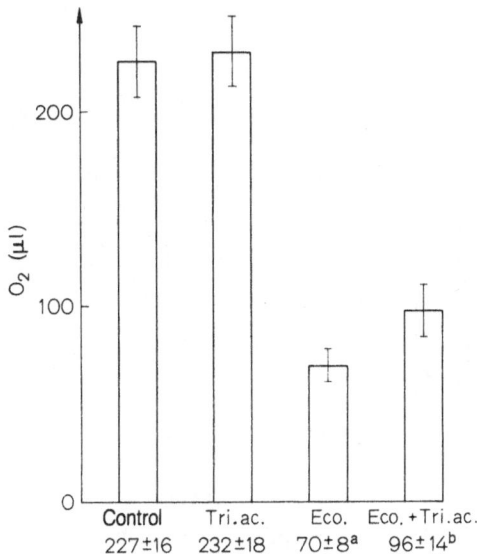

	Control	Tri.ac.	Eco.	Eco.+Tri.ac.
	227 ± 16	232 ± 18	70 ± 8^a	96 ± 14^b

Fig. 22. Oxygen consumption of resting *Candida albicans* under the influence of econazole nitrate with and without triamcinolone acetonide. Econazole nitrate concentration: 20 µg/ml, triamcinolone acetonide concentration: 1000 µg/ml; duration of test: 120 min; medium: Ringer glucose DMFA. ECO = econazole nitrate, TRI = triamcinolone acetonide. [a] $P < 0.001$ vs. control. [b] $P > 0.01$ vs. econazole nitrate alone

effect of isoconazole or econazole on *Staphylococcus aureus haemolyticus* in the resting or proliferating phase (at a steroid concentration up to 50 times the econazole concentration) [242].

It can be concluded from these results that the antimicrobial action of econazole nitrate is not inhibited by the presence of hydrocortisone or triamcinolone acetonide, provided the steroid concentration is not higher than the econazole concentration [239]. It remained to be determined how the presence of triamcinolone acetonide affects the *penetration* of econazole nitrate (see also Sect. 6.2.2).

Absorption studies after epicutaneous application to the skin of rabbits showed that absorption during the first few hours is reduced by the presence of triamcinolone acetonide. When viewed over longer periods of time, however, no effect on absorption is observed; that is, penetration is unchanged, and higher tissue levels of econazole must be assumed during the first few hours due to diminished absorption and removal via the circulation. Details of these test results are presented in Fig. 23 [52]. The diminished removal of econazole via the circulation may be attributed to the opening of the shunts and the associated decrease of blood flow through the papillary region as a result of the glucocorticoid action.

When two drugs are combined, it is of course necessary to rule out antagonistic interactions *in both directions*. Accordingly, the granuloma pouch test

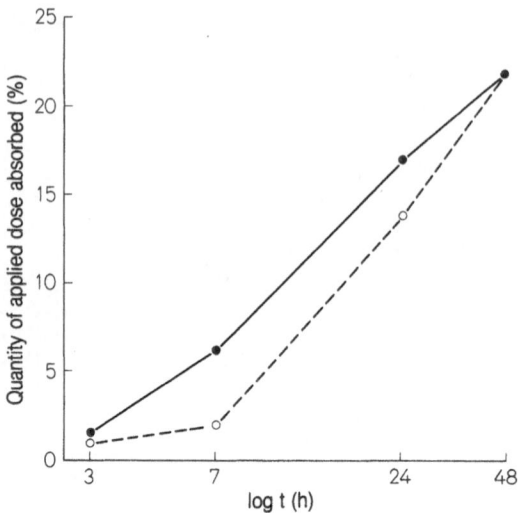

Fig. 23. Skin absorption of econazole nitrate (1%) (●—●) from a cream base in the rabbit. Comparison with absorption in the presence of triamcinolone acetonide (0.1%) (○---○). From data in [52].

was performed on rats to compare the quantity of exudate after application of triamcinolone acetonide alone with the quantity of exudate after application of triamcinolone acetonide combined with econazole nitrate. It was found that the antiexudative action (anti-inflammatory activity) of triamcinolone acetonide was not at all impaired by the imidazole derivative.

It also had to be determined whether the imidazole derivatives would interfere with the permeation and pharmacologic activity of glucocorticoids on human skin. This was investigated by means of the blanching phenomenon (details of method in [242]). Ethanolic steroid solutions were prepared in four different concentrations; a ten times higher concentration of econazole nitrate was added to a portion of the solutions. Then the percentage of the test sites that showed a marked blanching reaction after application of the steroid or the steroid/econazole solution was determined. The presence of econazole nitrate failed to influence the blanching reaction produced by triamcinolone acetonide. Such a test result is shown graphically in Fig. 24.

There is still no ideal test for assaying the external activities of glucocorticoids. The blanching phenomenon caused by opening of the shunts gives information only on the penetration of the glucocorticoid and on one pharmacologic activity which may not be very important clinically. However, it has been confirmed repeatedly [231] that a good correlation exists between the activity of various glucocorticoids in the blanching test and their therapeutic efficacy on external application. For the time being, or until a better model is developed, the pharmacologic testing of glucocorticoids for topical therapy is still best accomplished by eliciting the blanching phenomenon.

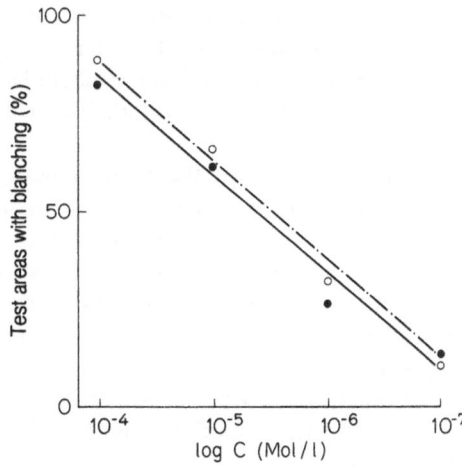

Fig. 24. The blanching phenomenon on human skin, elicited by triamcinolone acetonide in various concentrations (O–·–O). For comparison, triamcinolone acetonide with tenfold concentration of econazole nitrate (●—●). Data in % blanched areas (see [242])

Thus, it has been determined not only that the antimicrobial activity and penetration of econazole nitrate are not impaired by glucocorticoids in certain concentration ranges, but also that conversely the penetration and vascular action of the glucocorticoids are not significantly altered by econazole nitrate.

4.4.5 Antibacterial Substances

When econazole nitrate was combined with butirosin, an aminoglycoside antibiotic (10:3 ratio), no interference was observed; in the case of *Pseudomonas,* the activity of the antibiotic was enhanced by the presence of econazole nitrate, which is inactive against gram-negative organisms. Azidoamphenicol does not influence the antimycotic activity of clotrimazole [217].

4.4.6 Antimycotic Substances

It will never be necessary in *local therapy* to combine any of the imidazole derivatives with another antimycotic agent. The situation is different in the *systemic treatment* of fungal infections, however. Here the concurrent use of an imidazole antifungal and one of the polyene antibiotics may prove beneficial. It is reported, for example, that candidal sepsis responded well to the oral administration of miconazole, but candidal arthritis had to be treated adjunctively with intraarticular injections of amphotericin B [179].

In systemic therapy with miconazole and amphotericin B, the surprising discovery was made that the combination was less effective than the administration of a single component. This clinical observation prompted *in vitro* studies. It was found in these tests that the combination of miconazole (tested at 1–200 μg/ml) or econazole and amphotericin B (1–20 μg/ml) led to antagonistic effects in *Candida albicans* [80, 267]. Under no conditions, a synergism was seen [7].

Some tests dealt with the interactions of clotrimazole and econazole nitrate with amphotericin B, natamycin, and nystatin. The Warburg test on resting *Candida albicans* demonstrated an antagonistic interaction between the two groups of drugs with regard to antimycotic activity. The antibacterial activity, tested on *Staphylococcus aureus,* of imidazole derivatives (econazole, ketoconazole) decreased in the presence of polyene antibiotics (nystatin, amphotericin B) [244].

The antagonism between polyene antibiotics and imidazole derivatives may be based on various mechanisms. The action of the polyenes is developed in two phases:
1) Binding to sterols in the fungal cell membrane
2) Disturbance of cell permeability

Imidazole may interfere with either the binding phase or the creation of a permeability disturbance. On the other hand, it is possible that polyenes exert a protective action against imidazoles. A direct chemical reaction which yields an antimycotically inactive product is yet another possibility. It is noteworthy that both the imidazole derivatives and the polyenes are *lipid reactors;* both groups rarely lead to sensitization, which may have to do with their good lipid reactivity and poor protein reactivity (no complete-antigen formation) [233, 237]. Based on available test results, the combined use of an imidazole derivative and a polyene antibiotic (amphotericin B) is not recommended for practical clinical purposes. With fluorocytosine and econazole, a synergistic antifungal action was reported [80]. This observation could not be confirmed in Warburg experiments on resting yeasts (personal investigations).

4.4.7 Antibacterial Substances and Glucocorticoids

Preparations are used in veterinary medicine which contain imidazole derivatives in combination with butirosin and triamcinolone acetonide. The relative concentrations of these drugs are 10:3:1. Tests *in vitro* have shown that no antagonistic interactions take place in such combinations with regard to antimicrobial effectiveness. Also, clotrimazole is not influenced by azidoamphenicol or dexamethasone [217].

4.4.8 Conclusions

According to available test results, the antifungal imidazole derivatives can be used in the local treatment of skin and mucous membrane diseases with no fear of antagonistic interactions. While there are isolated reports that the activity of imidazoles is reduced by proteins, this reduction is too slight to be clinically relevant. It is also true that lipids present on the skin surface can inhibit the antimycotic action of econazole nitrate *in vitro,* but only in extremely high concentrations. In clinical usage, there is no danger that the activity of econazole will be impaired by skin-surface lipids.

If the combined application of imidazole dervatives and antibacterial antibiotics is indicated, there is no need to fear antagonistic interactions. Only the combined use of imidazoles and polyene antibiotics is not advised.

4.5 Bioavailability Studies

Information on the bioavailability of a drug is most valuable when based on clinical experiments and observations. In the case of antimicrobials, high drug concentrations must be attained at the site of infection over an extended period of time. Antimicrobials should therefore be somewhat difficult to remove from the skin surface. The drugs should penetrate into the skin, but they should not permeate the skin too well, lest they be removed too quickly by the vascular system. The determination of bioavailability for questions of external therapy is sometimes difficult. Available models usually introduce some degree of error. It is simple enough to measure drug concentrations at the skin surface, but this provides information only on the retention time and stability of the drug. It tells nothing about penetration.

The release of active drug from preparations for external therapy can be determined *in vitro;* it is assumed that the drug release occurs in a similar manner on the skin surface. The release of the drug from preparations must be tested, because if it is incorporated "too well" (too stable), its release may be hindered. Drug release can be easily determined by means of the Petri-dish agar diffusion test. Simulated membranes (lipid membranes, protein membranes) may then be used to test for drug penetration. The influence of galenic additives on bioavailability can be well demonstrated by the use of such models [86].

Next it is necessary to determine drug release when the preparation is applied to human skin. After a specified duration of action, skin layers are removed by stripping, or biopsies are performed. Detection of the drug is difficult due to the very low concentrations present in deeper layers, and so a radiolabeled drug is usually employed. Of course this shows only the penetration of "radioactivity," and not necessarily of active drug. But it does demonstrate that drug release from the preparation has transpired.

The degree of transcutaneous permeation can also be measured in the penetration chamber, but in this human skin (from corpses) should be used. Drug release and penetration into deeper layers of the human skin were also determined *in vivo* for the imidazole derivatives clotrimazole and econazole nitrate, using radiolabeled compounds. After external application in ointment or cream form to healthy or stripped skin, biopsies were performed, and the depth of penetration was determined from the presence of radioactive material (e. g., by autoradiography) [78, 270] (see Sects. 6 and 8 for more details).

Thus, the release of the imidazole derivatives from their corresponding external preparations has been established. It remains to be determined by chemical analysis or by the demonstration of clinical (therapeutic) efficacy whether the drugs are released in antimicrobially active form. Such investigations are first carried out on experimental animals.

5 Therapeutic Use of Imidazole Derivatives in Animals (Experimental Therapy)

5.1 Local Application

The demonstration of antimycotic activity *in vitro* does not necessarily mean that the drug can also be used for the treatment of mycoses in external therapy. For example, many polyene antibiotics (such as nystatin) exhibit activity against dermatophytes *in vitro,* but fail completely when tested for therapeutic efficacy against dermatophyte infections (see [233]).

Before a new antimycotic agent undergoes clinical tests on humans, it is first tested in animals. It is a simple matter to induce a *cutaneous infection* with dermatophytes in guinea pigs and rabbits. However, it is often difficult to induce candidosis of the skin. For example, guinea pigs must first be treated with toxic doses of chlortetracycline or with alloxan in order for a candidal infection to develop. Rabbits must usually be treated with glucocorticoids (suppression of immune response) before infection with *Candida albicans* can be achieved. *Vaginal* candidosis can be induced in rats by direct infection.

The therapeutic efficacy of the usual external preparations of imidazole derivatives (clotrimazole, miconazole nitrate, econazole nitrate) has been demonstrated in the models indicated. For example, two concentrations of econazole nitrate (2% and 0.5%) were compared with equal concentrations of tolnaftate in guinea pigs with experimentally induced trichophytosis *(Trichophyton mentagrophytes* or *Microsporum canis).* During *prophylactic* application (cream applied daily, starting on the day after infection), all four preparations were successful. The same finding was made during *curative* application: A clinical and microbiologic cure was effected in all animals within 3–6 weeks [110, 111, 309].

It was found that 1% and 2% econazole nitrate was just as successful in treating cutaneous candidosis in the guinea pig as nystatin or amphotericin B in the usual concentrations. Thus, the results of animal experiments provided justification for the use of imidazole derivatives in the treatment of cutaneous and mucocutaneous mycoses in man.

5.2 Systemic Application

A number of animal models are available for systemic mycoses and for the testing of systemic antimycotics. It has been shown in various animal species that the imidazole derivatives clotrimazole, miconazole, and econazole are suited for the systemic treatment of mycoses. For example, econazole proved just as effective as griseofulvin in the treatment of *guinea pig* trichophytosis when administered orally in doses of at least 160 mg/kg/day over a 14-day period. In experimental candidosis (see Sect. 5.1), econazole was also effective in low doses (10 or 40 mg/kg). (The ineffectiveness of the polyenes on oral administration was reaffirmed in this model.) Vaginal candidosis in *rats* was cured with econazole in doses of 80 and 160 mg/kg/day (administered by stomach tube over 14 days). The cultures were negative in all animals [309]. In *mice,* experimentally induced candidosis (*Candida albicans* injected into caudal vein) or aspergillosis *(Aspergillus niger)* always has a fatal outcome. By giving increasing amounts of the drug 2 h before injection of the fungi and then 4 and 24 h afterward, the minimum life-prolonging dose can be determined (oral and intraperitoneal administration). Econazole was practically ineffective against experimental candidosis (minimum life-prolonging dose above 200 mg/kg), while fluorocytosine had a marked effect beyond a dose of 25 mg/kg, and amphotericin B beyond a dose of 0.6 mg/kg. In another series of tests in which clotrimazole, miconazole, and econazole were given orally to mice infected intravenously with *Candida albicans,* clotrimazole proved superior to the other two imidazole derivatives at a dose of 100 mg/kg twice daily over a 5-day period. Miconazole had no significant influence on the survival rate. In still other series in mice, oral miconazole prevented and cured candidal infections of the gastrointestinal tract [310], an observation that led to its recommendation in humans for "fungal sterilization" before intestinal surgery. Clotrimazole achieved almost the degree of efficacy of amphotericin B (0.5 mg/kg per application) in this series of tests [110, 111].

In animals infected experimentally with *Aspergillus,* econazole exerted a life-prolonging effect in an oral dose of 100 mg/kg [188]. Against experimental cryptococcosis in mice, both miconazole and econazole (given orally or intramuscularly) were highly effective [163, 165]. Ketoconazole proved most effective upon oral administration in experimental coccidioidomycosis in mice [163, 164].

On the whole, the animal experiments confirm that the imidazole derivatives clotrinazole, econazole, miconazole, and ketoconazole exert a good antimycotic action when administered systemically. They can be given orally, intramuscularly, or intravenously. It should be noted that the activity of these drugs, especially clotrimazole, may be diminished during prolonged administration as a result of enzyme induction in the host organism (cf. Sect. 6.2.1).

6 General Pharmacology of the Imidazole Derivatives in Man and Animals

6.1 Pharmacologic Properties (Apart from Antimicrobial Action)

The antimicrobially active imidazole derivatives were investigated for their other pharmacologic properties in numerous screening tests. The results were entirely negative (no anti-inflammatory action, no effects on circulation, no central or autonomic nervous effects, no respiratory depression, no effect on α- or β-receptors, no anticholinergic action, no antiserotonin action).

An easily reversible binding to serum proteins takes place in the organism; numerous binding sites have been demonstrated.

The pure base of miconazole and econazole is intended for systemic application. The nitrates are used only in local therapy.

6.2 Absorption, Excretion, and Metabolism in Animals

6.2.1 Systemic Application

The imidazole derivatives clotrimazole, miconazole, econazole, and ketoconazole are absorbed when administered orally and can be detected in the serum. For example, a dose of 15 mg/kg *clotrimazole* produces serum levels up to 15 µg/ml [207]. The distribution of the imidazole derivatives in animals is practically the same after oral and intravenous administration.

Extensive studies have been done in rats, rabbits, dogs, and monkeys on the absorption, excretion, and metabolism of *econazole* following oral administration. The highest plasma level is achieved 4 h after oral ingestion. Rats and dogs manifest a very high elimination of econazole and its metabolites in the stool, regardless of whether the drug is administered orally or intravenously. This is indicative of a biliary excretion. The often very long bioactive half-lives of the drug (115 h for the blood in beagle dogs) suggest an enterohepatic circulation.

Only a slight amount of econazole was recovered unchanged from the stool and urine of the three animal species tested. Considerable differences in the distribution and excretion of econazole were observed in some cases between male and female animals.

The plasma levels and excretory values after oral administration of ^{3}H-labeled econazole nitrate in rats, dogs, and monkeys *(Macaca fasicularis)* are given in Table 9. The values were calculated on the basis of detected *radioactivity*. An identification of econazole nitrate itself was performed in the urine and stool [56]. Excreted metabolites are mostly glucuronides.

A workup of various animal organs failed to show any prevalence in terms of the deposition or metabolism of imidazole derivatives. Organs involved in the metabolism and excretion of foreign substances displayed a higher content.

The administration of econazole-^{14}C in monkeys basically confirmed the results obtained for econazole-^{3}H. After 8 h, a serum level of 1.8 µg/ml was achieved. Within 6 days, 55% of the administered dose (radioactivity!) was present in the stool and 29% in the urine.

Urine studies resulted in the detection of more than 20 metabolites of econazole. Five major metabolites and two minor metabolites were identified. More than 50% of the radioactivity present in the urine after administration of radiolabeled econazole is attributable to a reaction product formed by the splitting off the *p*-chlorobenzyl radical. The detection of these metabolites allows us to hypothesize on the metabolic transformation of econazole. One such hypothesis is illustrated in Fig. 25. The first step is the introduction of hydroxyl groups at the imidazole radical, followed by oxidative splitting of the imidazole ring. Further degradation is accompanied by the removal of CO_2 and NH_3 [60]. Note that both unchanged and metabolized econazole which contain the label (^{14}C or ^{3}H) are detected in tissue radioactivity studies. This must be taken into account when test results are evaluated.

It was again confirmed that the repeated administration of imidazole antimycotics leads to enzyme induction. This causes a much more rapid breakdown

Table 9. The fate of orally administered econazole-^{3}H in rats, monkeys, and dogs

	Rat male	female	Monkey male	female	Dog male	female
Highest plasma level (µg/ml)	10.1	6.0	6.2	5.5	6.5	8.3
Highest plasma level (% dose)	2.3	1.3	1.7	1.5	1.7	2.2
Highest plasma level (after h.)	2	4	4–8	4–8	<1	2
Radioactivity in the urine (% of dose)	24.3	17.3	57.6	47.4	15.7	27.1
Radioactivity in the feces (% of dose)	77.0	87.7	25.5	36.6	46.9	63.7
Unchanged econazole in the urine (% of dose)	4.2	4.3	9.0	4.6	1.4	2.1
Unchanged econazole in the feces (% of dose)	3.8	5.0	4.0	8.5	10.0	2.1

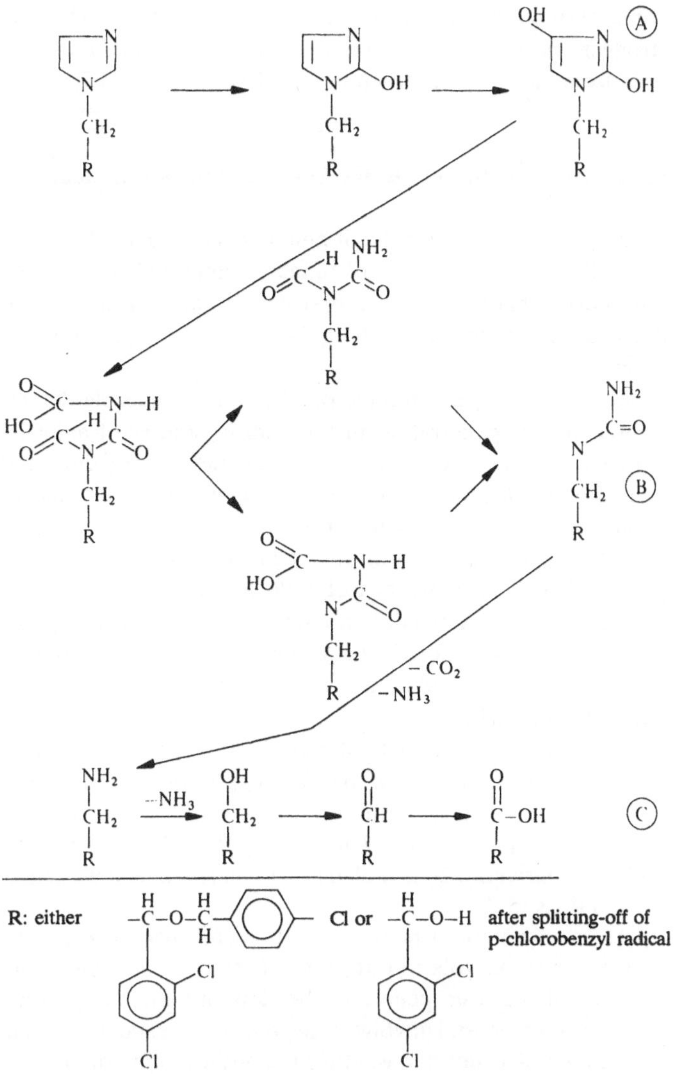

Fig. 25. Metabolic breakdown of the antimicrobially active imidazole derivatives. Illustration of a hypothesis based on metabolites detected after administration of econazole nitrate-^{14}C in monkeys. A and C = major metabolites of the degradation product, B = minor metabolite of econazole

of the drug, and therefore greatly reduces its clinical efficacy. Differences were found between different animal species with regard to enzyme induction. Clotrimazole caused the most marked enzyme induction in all the animal species; this property was confirmed in humans as well. Miconazole also produces a marked enzyme induction in experimental animals (comparable to that of clotrimazole); but in humans, this effect is slight. In dogs, clotrimazole produces a stronger enzyme induction than miconazole. So far, no enzyme induction by econazole has been observed in man (see [31, 76, 117]).

6.2.2 Local Application to the Skin and Mucous Membranes

When evaluating the results of animal experiments, it must be taken into account that the penetration of organic compounds through the skin varies in different animal species. The best penetration is achieved on rabbit skin and decreases from the rat to the guinea pig. The penetration rate is lowest for human skin.

On the whole, the antimicrobially active imidazole derivatives show good transcutaneous penetration in the various species of animals tested. For example, serum levels of 220 ng/ml (calculated from radioactivity) are achieved 24 h after application of 10 mg econazole nitrate ^{3}H to intact rabbit skin. After application to abraded skin, serum levels of 307 ng/ml are reached after 8 h. Absorption of a single drug depot on the skin surface requires 8 days. The presence of triamcinolone acetonide lowers the high blood levels obtained during the first 24 h, but does not influence the total absorption (Fig. 23). Tests on rabbit skin also showed that econazole nitrate is distributed through all the skin layers; no accumulation in a particular layer could be detected by micro-autoradiography [52].

About 30% of the dose of econazole nitrate applied to the *outer skin* of rabbits is absorbed. On *intravaginal application,* a total absorption of about 50% is achieved (dose: 5 mg econazole nitrate ^{3}H); the peak serum level of 307 ng/ml is obtained after 6 h. About 30% of the drug is absorbed from the rabbit *vagina* within 24 h, which is in good agreement with the results of similar tests in dogs [52].

Thus, animal experiments have also confirmed the penetration of imidazole derivatives (econazole nitrate) into the skin. In animals, comparatively larger amounts of the drug penetrate the skin and enter the serum. Of course the results presented still involve a degree of uncertainty: When radioactivity is determined, it is unclear whether the antimycotic drug is present in active or metabolized form.

6.3 Absorption, Excretion, and Metabolism in Man

6.3.1 Systemic Application

Clotrimazole, miconazole, econazole, and ketoconazole are absorbed when administered orally in humans (plasma level). As in laboratory animals, excretion is via the biliary route with the feces or via the kidneys with the urine.

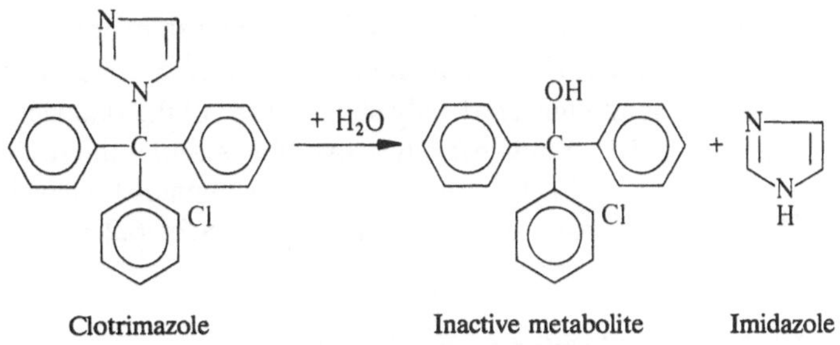

Clotrimazole   Inactive metabolite   Imidazole

Fig. 26. Hydrolytic splitting of clotrimazole in highly acidic solution (gastric juice)

Only 20 min after oral administration of 1.5 g *clotrimazole,* the drug or its metabolites can be detected in the serum. The highest level of 15 µg/ml is achieved after 3 h, again calculated by determination of radioactivity [79]. At higher doses (100 mg/kg/24 h), serum levels of 150 µg/ml can be calculated from the radioactivity [128]. Because the actual antimycotic activity does not correspond to this value, it must be assumed that radioactive metabolites with no antimicrobial activity are mainly responsible for this value.

Following the oral administration of *miconazole,* the peak serum levels are reached after about 2–4 h. The administration of 522 mg leads to serum levels of about 0.4 µg/ml; administration of a double dose produces peak values of 1.2 µg/ml [304]. By administering 500 mg every 8 h, serum levels of 0.95–1.75 µg/ml can be maintained [53].

The oral administration of 1 g *econazole* leads to a serum level of 0.9 µg/ml after 6 h [53]. Other authors report mean values of 1.25 µg/ml [55, 76]. Values measured at shorter intervals after oral administration were higher in some cases [244]; the peak value was 13 µg/ml (1 h after oral ingestion of acid-resistant capsules). The drug is absorbed in the small intestine [54].

When administered orally, imidazole derivatives should be given only in the form of acid-resistant capsules [82], for degradation will occur in a strongly acidic medium (gastric juice); the imidazole ring is hydrolytically split, as is shown for clotrimazole in Fig. 26.

Econazole is also administered to humans in the form of *intravenous* injections or infusions. A dose of 100 mg produces serum levels of 2.6 µg/ml within 15 min; the injection of 500 mg miconazole produces serum levels of 6 µg/ml [53]. Other authors report on the intravenous administration of econazole in doses of 200 and 400 mg, producing serum levels up to 8 µg/ml [76]. One oral dose of 0.2 g *ketoconazole* keeps up a serum level of 3 µg/ml.

The levels of imidazole derivatives detectable in the cerebrospinal fluid are only about one-tenth the plasma values [296]. Only very slight amounts are present in the saliva; concentrations up to 1.4 µg/ml occur in the pus.

The excretion of imidazole derivatives is by way of the bile and feces or via the kidneys. Renal damage does not significantly prolong the half-life of these drugs, indicating that biliary excretion is far more important than excretion in the urine [296].

Only a small amount of clotrimazole, miconazole, or econazole is excreted unchanged in the urine. It was shown in the case of miconazole that after the labeled drug is administered, only about 0.15% of the radioactivity is attributable to unchanged (antimicrobially active) miconazole; the rest consists of inactive metabolites [50]. Enzyme induction in humans by clotrimazole, miconazole, and econazole was already discussed in Sect. 6.2.1.

6.3.2 Local Application to the Outer Skin

Clotrimazole, miconazole nitrate, and econazole nitrate are applied to the skin of humans in 1% and 2% preparations. Under these conditions, not a single case of measurable antimycotic activity in the plasma has been discovered. When labeled substances are used, there is usually no measurable radioactivity in the plasma.

For example, *clotrimazole* (clotrimazole-^{14}C) applied in a 1% cream to 200 cm^2 skin surface in a dose of 800 mg produced no measurable radioactivity in the serum (8 test subjects). Less than 0.5% of the amount applied to the skin was detected in the urine over a 5-day period (calculated by radioactivity) [78].

In one study with human volunteers, *econazole nitrate* was more strongly absorbed than miconazole nitrate. Within 30 h, about 0.1% to 2% of the amount of econazole nitrate applied to the outer skin is excreted in the urine, depending on whether the skin was intact or stripped (labeled econazole nitrate was used in the tests). The urinary excretion corresponds rather closely to the amount reaching the deeper skin layers [270]. The skin levels of econazole nitrate will be discussed further in Sect. 8.

The serum levels and excretion of *miconazole nitrate* and *econazole nitrate* applied locally to intact and stripped skin are compared in Table 10. In the case

Table 10. Serum levels and excretion of miconazole nitrate [14]C (MICO) and econazole nitrate [14]C (ECO) after application to healthy normal and healthy stripped skin. Four subjects in each group. Judgment based on measured radioactivity. 1 g of a 2% cream was spread over 28 cm^2.

	Intact skin	Stripped skin
Mean value of highest plasma level	<1 ng/ml	MICO 8.4 ng/ml ECO 20 ng/ml
Time required to reach highest serum level	–	MICO 31 h ECO 18 h
Excretion in urine and feces (% of total dose)	MICO 0.02 ECO 0.1	MICO 1.1 ECO 3.7
Excretion in urine (% of total dose)	MICO 0.018 ECO 0.073	MICO 0.58 ECO 2.0
Excretion in feces (% of total dose)	MICO 0.004 ECO 0.029	MICO 0.49 ECO 1.7

of econazole nitrate, higher serum levels are achieved, the peak serum level is reached more quickly, and a higher percentage of the administered dose is excreted in the urine and feces. These results indicate a better penetration for econazole nitrate than for miconazole nitrate.

6.3.3 Local Application to the Vaginal Epithelium

The imidazole derivatives are absorbed more strongly after vaginal application than when applied to the skin. However, no antimycotic activity could be detected in the serum after the application of clotrimazole (100 mg in vaginal tablets), miconazole nitrate (5 g of a 2% cream), or econazole nitrate (5 g of a 1% cream or 50 mg in suppository form) [53].

It was determined by radiolabeling that about 1%–3% of the quantity of clotrimazole and miconazole nitrate introduced into the vagina is absorbed (measurement of radioactivity in the serum). For econazole nitrate, (by the same technique) absorption rates between 2.5% and 7% were measured [53, 202, 257, 325].

6.3.4 Conclusions

All imidazole derivatives are absorbed after oral administration. They should be given in the form of acid-resistant capsules. Therapeutically active serum levels can be achieved by intravenous injection, as has been impressively shown for econazole. Only with ketoconazole was oral administration (one tablet of 200 mg) able to maintain antifungally active serum levels.

The imidazole derivatives are also absorbed when applied locally to the skin and mucous membranes, but only to a slight degree; no systemic antimycotic activities are produced. The absorption of econazole nitrate is higher than that of clotrimazole and miconazole nitrate.

6.4 Sensitization

6.4.1 Preliminary Remarks

Drug allergies are among the most important problems of modern medicine. Drugs play a particularly important role as contact allergens: About 30% of all contact allergies are attributable to drug actions. As a result of experiences in recent decades, new drugs are now tested for their sensitizing capacity during the earliest phases of their development. This applies in particular to drugs for local use, for it is known that local application to inflamed skin areas entails a high risk of sensitization (see [247, 248] for further details).

The development of a drug allergy depends on three groups of factors. Sensitization-promoting *factors on the part of the drug* are primarily a high reactivity with proteins, for this promotes the formation of a complete antigen. The *site of application* also plays a role in sensitization; the application of drugs to the mucous membranes or to inflamed skin areas harboring microorganisms is particularly unfavorable. But antibiotics are devoutly used under these circumstances, which makes their sensitizing capacity especially important. The third group of factors involves the *disposition of the patient,* about which the least is known.

The final assessment of the sensitizing ability of a pharmacologic agent can be made only after years of clinical use. However, experimental investigations yield valuable clues and allow comparisons to be made with other substances already in clinical use.

The best animals for experimental investigations are rats and guinea pigs, although other species are also suitable. Testing a drug by *usage* is not recommended, because too many animals would be required. For example, if a sensitization index of 0.1% is considered acceptable, it would be necessary according to the laws of statistics to use the drug on 29,978 animals to be reasonably sure of obtaining a single case of sensitization [148]. Usage has also proved impractical in human subjects, for such large populations can be studied only in exceptional cases (e. g., mass prophylaxis).

The best alternative when investigating the sensitizing ability of a drug in man and animals is to employ *maximizing measures* [234, 236]. In *systemic* application, central and peripheral adjuvant effects should be utilized, and high concentrations employed. In *local* application, adjuvant effects should also be utilized, combined with damage to the cutaneous barrier. *Peripheral adjuvant effects* is a term referring to the stimulation of macrophages (formation of "angry" macrophages) by damage to their lysosomes, with a resultant decrease in the breakdown of phagocytized potential allergens. Associated with this is an increased transfer of allergens in (stimulating) form to the immune system.

Central adjuvant effects involve a nonspecific stimulation of the proliferation of preselected cell clones, which is manifested in a heightened readiness for antibody production (see [234] for further details).

6.4.2 Animal Experiments in Systemic Sensitization

Some tests have been done to determine whether guinea pigs and rats can be sensitized to econazole nitrate by the use of maximizing measures. On 2 successive days, 20 rats and 20 guinea pigs each received by intraperitoneal injection 400 mg econazole nitrate suspended in 0.15 mol/liter NaCl together with 0.5 ml of Freund's complete adjuvant. Fourteen days later the animals received 0.05 ml of a 0.1% econazole nitrate solution by intracutaneous injection. On the 15th day, 400 mg/kg was again administered intraperitoneally. Not a single experimental animal exhibited positive intracutaneous tests or shock reactions which would have indicated that sensitization had occurred. An allergy to human albumin could be induced in the overwhelming majority of the animals by employing the same technique.

6.4.3 Animal Experiments in Local Sensitization

Further series of tests were done to determine whether a delayed-type allergy to econazole nitrate could be induced in guinea pigs by maximizing measures, as by the method of Levine (using the drug in a mixture of ethanol, methyl Cellosolve and Tween 80) or by the method of Ehrmann and Raab (barrier damage by scarification, applying the drug together with Freund's complete adjuvant) (see [236]). All experiments in this direction failed. However, 21 of 50 guinea pigs could be sensitized to penicillin, and 27 of 40 animals sensitized to sulfanilamidothiazole by the methods indicated [236]. Sensitization to erythromycin could not be achieved (Table 11). Thus, it can be concluded from tests on laboratory animals that econazole does not exert a sensitizing action, at least to any degree which is relevant for external therapy.

6.4.4 Sensitization in Man

Clotrimazole, as well as miconazole nitrate and econazole nitrate, have been used for some years in the external treatment of mycotic infections of the skin and mucous membranes in man. To date, only three cases of hypersensitivity to miconazole have been documented [263, 344] as well as two cases of an allergy to clotrimazole [33, 259].

6.5 Anaphylactoid Activity

Many pharmacologic agents possess anaphylactoid activity; that is, they are capable either of releasing histamine from mast cells (anaphylactoid activity of the cellular type) or of activating kinins from their precursors (serum or tissue globulins) (anaphylactoid activity of the humoral type). In local therapy, such effects may be marked by an unpleasant burning, especially in the presence of barrier damage as may occur in cases of severe inflammation.

The clinical pictures of anaphylactoid ("anaphylaxis-like") and allergic phenomena of the immediate type are similar. The main pathogenic difference is that in allergic reactions the release of histamine (or activation of kinins) occurs as the result of an antigen-antibody reaction. In anaphylactoid reactions, no antibodies are present, and histamine release or kinin activation is the result of a dose-dependent pharmacologic response. Table 12 gives a comparison between local allergic and anaphylactoid reactions and the methods available for differentiating them.

Table 11. Experimental sensitization of guinea pigs in maximizing test to certain antimicrobial drugs important in local therapy [236]

Drug	Total number of animals	Number of animals sensitized
Na-Penicillin-G	50	21
Sulfanilamidothiazole	40	27
Erythromycin	35	0
Econazole nitrate	50	0

Table 12. Comparison of local allergic and anaphylactoid reactions (cellular anaphylactoid reactions)

	Allergic	Anaphylactoid
Reaction on initial contact	−	+
Latency after initial contact	+	−
Presence of antibodies (immediate reactions) or immune cells (delayed reactions)	+	−
Concentration- or dose-dependent intensity of reaction	−	+
Epicutaneous tests with *low* concentrations	+	−
Epicutaneous tests with *high* concentrations	+	+ or −[a]
Epicutaneous tests under occlusion on stripped skin with higher concentrations	+	+
Intracutaneous tests with *low* concentrations	+	−
Intracutaneous tests with *high* concentrations	+	+[b]
Clinical and histologic picture	identical	
Tachyphylaxis	+	+

[a] Redness, swelling.
[b] Also inflammatory, nodular delayed reaction in intracutaneous tests!

Among the antibiotics and chemotherapeutic agents for local application, there are a number of substances with cellular-type anaphylactoid activity [234]. In many cases there is a striking parallel between the basicity of a substance and its anaphylactoid activity. Table 13 lists the most important antimicrobials for local use together with their nitrogen content. Based on nitrogen content, the imidazole derivatives would be expected to have a lower anaphylactoid activity than neomycin. The detection of the anaphylactoid activity of neomycin in various models has been reported elsewhere [234].

In some studies econazole nitrate was compared with neomycin in the *dye displacement test* and the *rat mast-cell degranulation test* — two classic methods for the quantitative assessment of cellular-type anaphylactoid activity.

Table 13. Nitrogen content of some locally applied antimicrobials

Substance	Molecular weight	Number of nitrogen atoms	% Nitrogen
Neomycin (s)	774	8	15
Gentamicin	450	5	15
Chlormidazole	263	2	11
Clotrimazole	345	2	8
Miconazole nitrate			
Isoconazole nitrate	479	3	9
Miconazole (base)			
Isoconazole (base)	416	2	7
Econazole nitrate	445	3	9
Econazole (base)	382	2	7
Chlorquinaldol	228	1	6
Clioquinol	305	1	6
Haloprogin	361	–	–
Triclosan	290	–	–

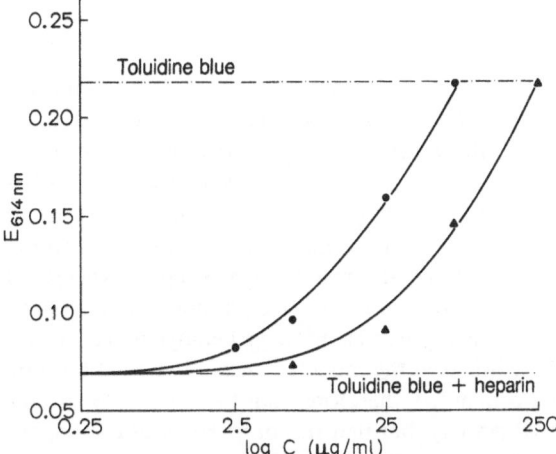

Fig. 27. *Comparative study of econazole nitrate* (▲—▲) *and neomycin* (●—●) *in the dye displacement test.* As the drug concentration increases, an increasing amount of toluidine blue is released from the toluidine blue – heparin complex; the absorption at 614 nm increases (after [237])

The classic *dye displacement test* is based on the splitting of the metachromatic heparin – toluidine blue complex by anaphylactoid substances. As increasing amounts of anaphylactoid substances are added, the intrinsic color of the toluidine blue becomes increasingly pronounced (measurement at 614 nm, the absorption peak of toluidine blue). The results of the dye displacement test are shown in Fig. 27: The absorption at 614 nm increases with increasing

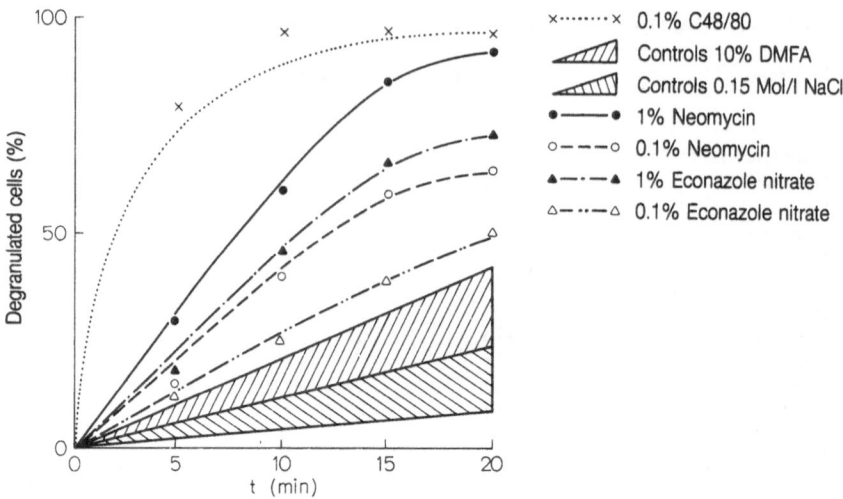

Fig. 28. *The degranulation of surviving rat mast cells by neomycin and econazole nitrate as a function of exposure time.* Neomycin was dissolved in 0.15 mol/l NaCl, econazole nitrate in 10% dimethyl formamide (after [237])

amounts of neomycin or econazole nitrate. The anaphylactoid activity of econazole nitrate is about one-tenth the anaphylactoid activity of neomycin.

In the *rat mast-cell degranulation test,* suspensions of surviving peritoneal mast cells are mixed with drug solutions in various concentrations. The mast cells are morphologically assessed after 5, 10, 15, and 20 min, and the percentage of degranulated mast cells is determined (for details see [232, 247, 248]). Fig. 28 shows the results of a comparative test of neomycin and econazole nitrate in the rat mast-cell degranulation test. Again, econazole nitrate is seen to be clearly less active than neomycin. The investigation of other imidazole derivatives in the models indicated yielded essentially the same results. It can be concluded, therefore, that the imidazole antifungals possess an anaphylactoid activity, but that this property does not impair the usefulness of the imidazole derivatives in 1%–2% topical preparations. However, it is still important that the presence of such a property be known; for if an allergy to an imidazole derivative is suspected, patch tests with excessive concentrations of the drug (as was done for neomycin!) would create the false impression of a positive test through anaphylactoid effects. The anaphylactoid activity of the imidazole derivatives explains why their application to acute lesions sometimes produces a burning sensation, caused by the release of histamine.

7 Toxicology of the Imidazole Derivatives

7.1 Preliminary Remarks

Although the antimicrobially active imidazole derivatives (with the exception of ketoconazole) are now used almost exclusively for local therapy, it is nevertheless important that their toxicological properties be known. One need only consider the accidental ingestion of external preparations by children.

The imidazole derivatives are relatively nontoxic. In laboratory animals, symptoms of intoxication appear only after high doses are administered. Like the polyene antibiotics, the imidazole derivatives act at the surfaces of cells and subcellular structures. This naturally raises the question of whether the imidazoles are active hemolytically. However, concentrations between 10 and 150 $\mu g/ml$ fail to produce hemolysis in human erythrocytes. This contrasts with the hemolytic effects of the sterol-reactive polyene antibiotics, for human erythrocyte membranes contain sterols with which the polyenes can react.

7.2 Systemic Toxicity

The relatively low toxicity of the imidazole derivatives is illustrated by the following LD_{50} values of econazole for various animal species and various modes of administration:

Mouse: 520 $\pm$ 70 mg/kg orally, 370 $\pm$ 43 mg/kg intraperitoneally, over 1600 mg/kg subcutaneously, 113 $\pm$ 5 mg/kg intravenously.

Rat: 920 $\pm$ 80 mg/kg orally, 315 $\pm$ 39 mg/kg intraperitoneally, over 1600 mg/kg subcutaneously, 49 $\pm$ 1 mg/kg intravenously.

Guinea pig: 252 $\pm$ 13 mg/kg orally.

In the *dog* and *monkey,* the oral administration of more than 200 mg/kg econazole induces vomiting, and so no oral LD_{50} can be determined. The intravenous administration of econazole in a dose of 35 mg/kg was lethal in 25% of the animals tested (dogs). Death was accompanied by signs of central nervous stimulation with an elevation of muscle tone and tonic-clonic spasms (membrane action?).

The determination of the LD_{50} of ready-to-use preparations containing imidazole derivatives yielded no new information. The oral LD_{50} of a 1% econazole nitrate cream is equal to 51 g/kg; that of the vehicle is 115 g/kg (rat).

In tests conducted to determine subacute and chronic toxicity, no specific toxic effects were found. The imidazole derivatives proved to be nonmutagenic, nonteratogenic, and nonembryotoxic in low, clinically relevant doses [31, 308]. Clotrimazole was reported to cause enzyme induction, while other imidazole derivatives caused liver enlargement and hepatic enzyme changes in animals. In man, however, no enzyme induction was produced by the systemic administration of econazole, as previously indicated [76].

7.3 Local Toxicity

7.3.1 Skin and Mucous Membrane Tolerance in Animals

The long-term use of external imidazole preparations (1%, 2%) in rabbits and dogs led to no local or systemic pathological changes. In 1% preparations, all imidazole derivatives were well tolerated when applied to the rabbit eye. Tests of the vaginal tolerance of imidazole derivatives in cream or suppository form showed good tolerance in all cases; no pathological symptoms were evident.

7.3.2 Photosensitizing Reactions

The tendency of a drug to produce photoallergic or phototoxic effects on local application can be predicted by testing *in vitro*.

If a drug is irradiated *in vitro* and its absorption spectrum is shifted toward longer wavelengths, it is likely that photoallergic effects will occur (sulfonamides, halogenated salicylanilides). On the other hand, if decoloration occurs (shift of absorption spectrum toward shorter wavelengths), the possibility of phototoxic effects must be considered. The same is true if a drug accelerates photochemical transformations (e. g., of benzophenone in isopropyl alcohol to benzopinacol and acetone) during irradiation, as has been demonstrated for porphyrins, furocumarines and tetracyclines [134].

Solutions of the imidazole derivatives (clotrimazole, miconazole nitrate, econazole nitrate) were found to be completely stable when irradiated *in vitro*. This precludes the occurrence of phototoxic or photoallergic reactions (see Sect. 8). In animal experiments, too, the external application of imidazole derivatives and subsequent irradiation produced no photosensitizing effects.

7.3.3 Skin and Mucous Membrane Tolerance in Man

In man, 1% and 2% preparations of the imidazole derivatives were found to be excellently tolerated by the skin. These concentrations can be applied several times daily without concern. Patients with known contact allergies also tolerate the imidazole derivatives very well; no inflammatory reactions were observed even under patch-test conditions, thus ruling out cross-allergies with known contact allergens. Such allergies would be unlikely in any case, owing to the novel chemical structure of the imidazoles.

The imidazole derivatives are not well tolerated in higher concentrations. For example, the application of 3% econazole nitrate preparations caused irritation in 6% of the persons tested. This increased to 11% in skin-sensitive subjects [299, 300]. Five-percent preparations are tolerated even less by the skin. This is probably due to the anaphylactoid activity of the imidazole derivatives (see Sect. 6.5). From this aspect, preference might be given to those preparations for external use which contain imidazole derivatives in a 1% concentration, as long as equal therapeutic efficacy is guaranteed (cf. Sect. 12).

Creams with a drug content of 1% and 2% as well as suppositories with 50, 100, or 150 mg of the drug are excellently tolerated by the vaginal mucosa. The tolerance is just as good as that of the vehicles employed, as shown in double-blind studies.

8 Clinical Pharmacology of Topical Antimicrobials with Special Regard to the Imidazole Derivatives

8.1 Preliminary Remarks

Microbial infections are on the increase in all branches of medicine. This is especially true of mycotic infections (for details, see Sect. 9 and 10). This increase is attributable in part to iatrogenic causes. Paradoxically, antimicrobial agents can lead to or promote microbial infections.

The increase in microbial infections has intensified the search for ever newer drugs to combat them. At present, a variety of highly effective substances are available. The selection of a specific agent is not based on efficacy alone, however. Considerations from the standpoint of the clinical pharmacologist are playing an increasingly important role [240]. In this chapter we shall discuss the general requirements placed by the clinical pharmacologist on drugs for local use. This will be followed by a look at the special requirements placed on antimicrobial drugs, and finally by a discussion of their preparation.

8.2 Physical Properties

Drugs for external use should be colorless and odorless. They should be stable when exposed to light (see Sect. 7.3.2 and 8.5). The physical properties of a drug further influence its usefulness in external preparations (see Sect. 3.3 and 8.11).

8.3 Skin Tolerance

Drugs for external use must be well tolerated by the skin, even when severe inflammation is present. The excellent skin and mucous membrane tolerance of the imidazole derivatives in 1% and 2% preparations, plus their favorable physical properties, make them well suited for external therapy. Used in low concentrations, they produce no unpleasant symptoms resulting from anaphylactoid effects.

If the permeability of the skin is increased (loosening of epidermis, damage to barrier) and if the degranulative tendency of the mast cells in the dermal connective tissue is elevated, even drugs with a weak anaphylactoid activity can induce histamine release. This causes a flare-up of the inflammation, with burning, and itching.

It is clear that the anaphylactoid activity of the imidazole derivatives (see Sect. 6.5) does not hamper their clinical usefulness. Otherwise the drug neomycin, whose anaphylactoid activity is about ten times greater, could not be used so frequently and successfully in external therapy.

8.4 Sensitization

From an allergological standpoint, locally applied antimicrobials are used under highly unfavorable conditions. Contact between the chemical substance and the patient takes place in the presence of microbes (adjuvant effects, see [234, 237]) as well as degenerative and inflammatory changes (see Sect. 6.4.1).

Experience has shown that drugs used locally on the skin and mucous membranes exhibit the highest sensitization rates [247]. It is for this reason that sulfonamides and penicillins are no longer used in local therapy (see Sect. 1.3 and 2). Antibiotics are becoming increasingly less important in local therapy, due to rising sensitization rates and the growing resistance of microorganisms. The macrolide antibiotics with a polyene structure may well be the only exception in this regard, for only a few cases of sensitization have been reported for these compounds. On the other hand, a nonmacrolide tetraene antibiotic, variotin, frequently leads to sensitization [199].

Series of tests in animals (see Sect. 6.4), clinical trials and years of clinical experience have all shown that the imidazole derivatives clotrimazole, miconazole nitrate, and econazole nitrate are practically *nonallergenic*. This fact is particularly noteworthy in view of the frequency of sensitization in local antimicrobial therapy (see Sect. 6.4.4).

8.5 Photosensitizing Reactions

Drugs for local use on the outer skin should produce neither photoallergic nor phototoxic reactions. The etiology of phototoxic and photoallergic reactions is shown schematically in Table 14.

Table 14. Phototoxic and photoallergic reactions due to antimicrobial substances

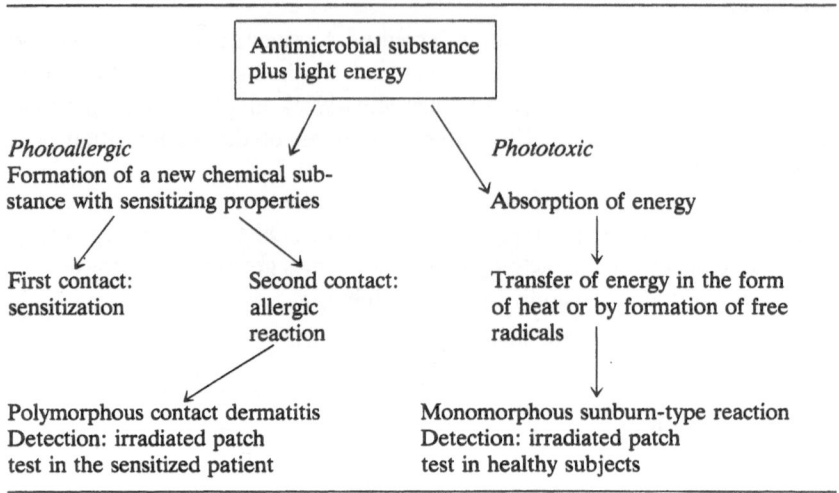

In each case, undesired reactions to visible or ultraviolet light arise from a change in the administered drug upon exposure to light (sunlight). In one case a new, strongly sensitizing compound if formed; in the other case, energy is absorbed and transmitted to skin cells.

Photosensitizing reactions can be ruled out during the use of imidazole derivatives. Clotrimazole, miconazole nitrate, and econazole nitrate remain stable (i. e., undergo no changes) on exposure to visible or ultraviolet light (see Sect. 7.3.2).

8.6 Interactions with Substances on the Skin Surface

Drugs for external use should retain their therapeutic efficacy in the presence of substances on the skin surface. The imidazole derivatives possess a protein reactivity, but it is very slight (see Sect. 4.4.2). They are antagonized by lipids only when the latter are present in very large amounts. Under the conditions of dermatologic therapy, antagonistic interactions with skin-surface lipids and proteins can be ruled out (see Sect. 4.4.3).

8.7 Penetration and Absorption

The ideal drug for local application would be one which penetrates well, but is not absorbed. Thus, a good penetrating ability into deeper skin layers is required, but absorption and removal by the vascular system should be avoided. Such a requirement cannot be fulfilled in practice.

However, it is important for antimicrobial drugs in particular to possess good penetration that will ensure active concentrations even in deeper skin layers. The need for antimicrobially active concentrations in deeper layers makes the use of substances with high minimum inhibitory concentrations (e. g., salicylic acid with inhibitory concentrations between 2 and 3 mg/ml [272]) as antimicrobials extremely problematic.

It has been shown that when clotrimazole and econazole nitrate are applied to the skin, microbicidal concentrations are achieved in the deeper layers of the epidermis, and microbistatic concentrations in the corium (Table 15). The values indicated were calculated by the use of radiolabeled imidazole derivatives [78, 207, 269, 270]. In the case of econazole nitrate, it could also be shown that the substance present in the deeper skin layers consists of antimicrobially active drug, and not inactive metabolites [268].

Isoconazole nitrate appears to range between clotrimazole and econazole nitrate in its dermal penetration. In the epidermis, concentrations of about 20 µg/ml were obtained after applying 5 mg of a cream containing 50 µg of the drug per square cm human skin (skin from corpses, experiments *in vitro*); in the dermal layers, concentrations of about 3 µg/ml were measured. The combined application of isoconazole nitrate with a glucocorticoid (diflucortolone-21-valerate or fluocortine butyrate) provoked an increase in the epidermal and dermal concentrations of isoconazole as shown in experiments on rabbit skin in vivo [306a].

Considering the importance of achieving antimicrobially active concentrations in deeper skin layers, it is little wonder that econazole is recognized as the prime product from the series of imidazole derivatives used in local therapy: This substance exhibits the highest antimicrobial activity and the best penetration (see Sect. 3.4.3 and 6.3). When applied in a varnish, econazole can even penetrate into an infected – not into a healthy – nail [268]; concentrations of about 400 µg/ml tissue are reached [268]. This good penetration is naturally accompanied by a higher absorption. The absorption of econazole and its metabolites is also higher than that of the other imidazole derivatives (see Sect. 6.3).

Penetration and absorption are higher in the presence of inflammatory or degenerative skin changes than on healthy skin. When applied therapeutically, the imidazole derivatives produce antifungal and antibacterial concentrations in the deeper skin layers. This explains the high therapeutic efficacy of the imidazole derivatives even in long-standing cases which have not responded to other antimicrobials.

Table 15. Concentrations of clotrimazole and econazole nitrate in various skin layers following the topical application of 1% preparations (after [207, 270])

Skin layer	Depth mm	Clotrimazole μg/ml	Econazole nitrate μg/ml
Stratum corneum	–	1000	1000
Barrier zone	0.05	200	200
Rete Malpighi	0.1	30	50
Stratum basale	0.2	20	25
Upper dermis	0.3	10	8
Middle dermis	0.6	2	4
Lower dermis	1.0	–	0.3

8.8 Systemic Administration

Drugs for local application should not be administered systemically, and vice versa. Of course this rule pertains only to drugs which lead to sensitization. If a patient is sensitized by the local administration of a drug, the subsequent systemic administration of the same or chemically similar drug can trigger a severe allergic reaction. For this reason the drug-registering authorities in many countries make a strict distinction between antibiotics for systemic use and antibiotics for local use.

Clotrimazole, miconazole, and econazole are intended primarily for use in local therapy. They are practically nonsensitizing (see Sect. 8.4) and are given systemically only in exceptional cases (see Sect. 11). Thus, the allergologist need have no second thoughts about using the imidazole derivatives in local therapy.

8.9 Use in Veterinary Medicine and the Food Industry

There are two reasons why drugs for human use are prohibited from use in veterinary medicine or the food industry: First, meat, milk, and other foods should not cause sensitizations or trigger allergic reactions; second, certain antimicrobials should be reserved exclusively for medicinal use so that the development of pathogen resistance will not be hastened by the widespread use of the substances.

The first consideration does not apply to the imidazole derivatives because they are practically nonsensitizing. The second consideration pertains mainly to the antibiotics. In the case of the imidazoles, the resistance level of bacteria and fungi has not changed since the introduction of these drugs nearly 10 years ago (see Sect. 4.3). Hence, there is no reason why imidazole derivatives should not be used in veterinary medicine – as is rearely done, cf. [213] – or in the food industry.

8.10 Special Clinical Pharmacologic Considerations in the Local Application of Antimicrobials

8.10.1 General

We have already discussed some of the requirements placed by the clinical pharmacologist on drugs for local use. These requirements also apply to local antimicrobials, of course. The requirements of good tolerance and low sensitization rate should be particularly emphasized. As mentioned earlier, infected lesions pose an extremely high risk of flare-up rections and sensitization. In addition to the requirements previously discussed, there are several special points to be considered during the local use of antimicrobials.

8.10.2 Degree and Spectrum of Activity

Antimicrobials for local use must demonstrate activity *in vivo,* under practical therapeutic conditions. Moreover, these drugs must possess a very high activity (low minimum inhibitory concentration), since the drug concentrations achieved in deeper skin layers are usually quite low (see Sect. 8.7). This requirement is satisfied by the imidazole derivatives. There is much debate about which type of antimicrobial spectrum is optimal for local therapy. It is often argued that drugs with a very narrow, specific action against a certain type of microorganism are the most suitable, for they do not upset the microbial balance too greatly and thus avoid adverse effects from the overgrowth of other strains. This is undoubtedly a valid line of reasoning. However, narrow-spectrum antimicrobials can be used only if the pathogenic microorganism is known, and only if one type of microorganism is present in the lesion. In many cases the microorganism can be identified with some degree of certainty from the clinical picture and by the direct examination of clinical preparations, but this usually reveals only the *predominant* infecting organism; mixed infections often occur (see Sect. 9.4). A reliable microbiological diagnosis (fungi and/or bacteria; different fungal strains) can be made only on the basis of time-consuming culture studies.

By direct examination alone, it cannot be determined whether dermatophytes or yeasts are present (see Sect. 10). For the reasons indicated, efforts are being directed more and more toward the use of antimycotics with broad activity. Today, drugs which are reliably active against all fungi pathogenic to man are preferred in local therapy. They are used in order to prevent therapeutic failure in case the clinical picture and direct microscopic findings are misleading. It should again be emphasized in this regard that the imidazole derivatives clotrimazole, miconazole nitrate, and econazole nitrate are active against all fungi pathogenic to man.

The demand for broad-spectrum antimycotics is particularly justified in cases of double infections or multiple coexisting infections caused by different types of fungi. The physician must always endeavor to prescribe only *one* preparation for his patient, even if multiple lesions are present.

Long-standing fungal infections are regularly colonized by bacteria (staphylococci). This is true of dermatophytoses as well as candidoses. Even if the staphylococci cannot be incriminated as the primary causative agents in such cases, they still contribute to the clinical symptoms and perpetuation of the lesion. Drugs which are active against fungi *and* staphylococci will lead to a faster and more reliable cure. At the same time, it has been proved that the metabolic products of certain fungus strains promote the growth and pathogenicity of staphylococci (see above). Conversely, staphylococci promote the growth and pathogenicity of various fungus strains (see Sect. 9 for details).

These circumstances have placed another requirement on the activity of broad-spectrum antimycotics: They should also be active against staphylococci. Activity against gram-negative organisms appears to be less important, because these bacteria are of little consequence as skin surface pathogens (see Sect. 9).

One should not gain the impression that the local administration of broad-spectrum antimicrobials leads to a type of sterilization of skin and mucous membrane surfaces. Only the numbers of the microorganisms are reduced. However, truly pathogenic strains are completely displaced — an effect due in large measure to the return of normal skin-surface saprophytes.

In addition to their broad antifungal spectrum, the imidazole derivatives clotrimazole, miconazole nitrate, and econazole nitrate also exhibit activity against gram-positive bacteria, and thus against staphylococci.

In the field of gynecology, drugs for the treatment of vaginitis should be active against gram-positive bacteria, yeasts, and trichomonads. The imidazole derivatives satisfy these requirements.

8.10.3 Resistance and Tolerance

It is seldom possible to test pathogen resistance in cultures before local treatment is administered. Treatment must be begun, at least, before such tests can be evaluated. Hence, *reliably effective* antimicrobials are preferred in order to minimize the problem of pathogen resistance.

This requirement is fulfilled by the imidazole derivatives. To date, no strain of microorganism with primary resistance to these drugs has been discovered (see Sect. 4.3).

8.11 Clinical Pharmacology of the Preparation

8.11.1 General

The physician is obliged during local therapy to administer the drug of choice in vehicles which are appropriate in terms of localization, of the lesion, of the stage of the disease and of the skin type. For this reason every drug should be offered in several forms (ointment, cream, lotion, powder, tincture).

For all galenic formulations of a drug, it must be shown that the drug is present in active, stable form and is released into the infected tissues under the conditions of external therapy (bioavailability). All topical preparations must show their expiration date.

Galenic formulations contain not only the drug and vehicle, but other ancillary ingredients, notably preservatives. Such ingredients are necessary in all but a few cases (self-stabilizing bases). Because the preservative-free bases developed in the past have not always been well tolerated, there is now a trend back to the use of preservatives.

The preservatives and emulsion stabilizers in dermatologic preparations are undoubtedly a source of sensitivity and hypersensitivity reactions in some cases, but this problem has been exaggerated. NIPA esters (parabens), for example, are now so widely used in cosmetics throughout the world that they are the second most abundant ingredient (next to water) contained in cosmetic products [168].

The *complete declaration* of all the ingredients of external preparations is essential. First, adverse reactions can be avoided if sensitivities or hypersensitivities to the preservatives or other ingredients in galenic preparations are known; and second, the pathogenesis of any adverse reactions that occur during therapy can be quickly ascertained.

8.11.2 Interactions

Preparations for external application consist of the drug, base, and ancillary ingredients. Interactions between these components which hamper the activity of the drug must be ruled out. This is usually done at an early stage, during the bioavailability testing of the drug.

Clinical circumstances sometimes make it advisable that preparations containing more than one drug be employed. In no case should a simple magistral mixture be given (mixture of two different preparations; incorporation of a second drug into an external preparation). The efficacy desired by the therapist would no longer be present in such a case.

Among the drug combinations most commonly used in external therapy are preparations which contain an antimicrobial and a glucocorticoid. These combinations are dealt with in the following section.

8.11.3 Combination of Imidazole Derivatives and Glucocorticoids

The first question to be asked with regard to the combined use of antimicrobials and glucocorticoids is whether antagonistic interactions take place *in vitro* or *in vivo*.

The possible interactions between these drugs and the possibility of ruling them out were discussed earlier (see Sect. 4.4.4). For example, econazole nitrate can be applied together with triamcinolone acetonide (10:1 ratio) without hesitation: The antimicrobial activity and penetration of the imidazole derivative are as little impaired as the penetration and activity of the glucocorticoid [52, 242]. The presence of higher concentrations of steroid would be unfavorable.

The second question to be answered concerns the behavior of skin-surface microorganisms on exposure to a combination of antimicrobial and glucocorticoid. Studies in this area are already available: Human skin was infected with *Staphylococcus aureus* or *Candida albicans,* and then a neomycin/gramicidin/nystatin/triamcinolone acetonide preparation was applied under occlusion. Afterwards, the microorganisms were counted (Table 16). The studies showed that the presence of glucocorticoids did not hamper the antimicrobial effectiveness of the antibiotics. Tests with staphylococci indicate that the presence of glucocorticoid alone leads to an increase in the number of microorganisms compared with test sites treated only with base [175]. This effect is the result either of a suppression of the body's defenses against infection, or of a direct stimulation of bacterial metabolism [231] – for glucocorticoids in *low* concentrations stimulate the metabolism of *Staphylococcus aureus* and *Candida albicans,* as well as of *Pseudomonas aeruginosa* (Fig. 29). The marked rise in the

Table 16. Pharmacologic studies on the effect of glucocorticoids on the activity of antibiotics applied locally to human skin (after [175])

Pretreatment	Organisms/cm^2
1. Infection with *Candida albicans*	
Nystatin and triamcinolone acetonide	0
Nystatin alone	0
Triamcinolone acetonide alone	16630
Vehicle	29560
No treatment	16470
2. Infection with *Staph. aureus*	
Neomycin/gramidicin and triamcinolone acetonide	80000 (10 of 13 lesions sterile)
Neomycin/gramicidin alone	20000 (8 of 13 lesions sterile)
Triamcinolone acetonide alone	40×10^6
Vehicle	24×10^6
No treatment	25×10^6

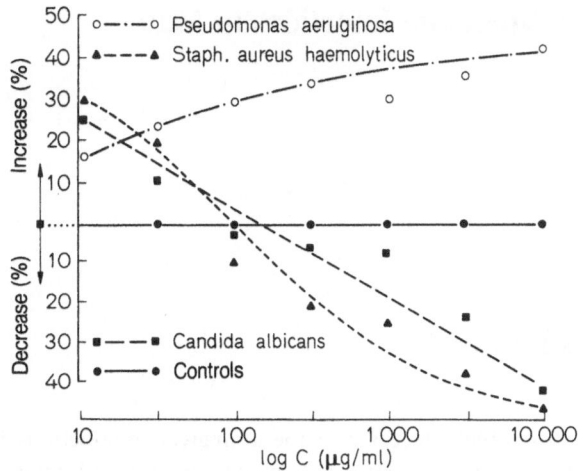

Fig. 29. *Oxygen consumption of resting bacteria or yeasts* under the influence of glucocorticoids (water-soluble glucocorticoid esters) in various concentrations

metabolic activity of the pseudomonads with increasing glucocorticoid concentrations is due to the metabolism of the ester part (succinate) of the steroid.

Although the presence of the glucocorticoid in these tests led to an increase in the number of microorganisms under occlusive dressings, only a very slight clinical response was observed. A severe inflammatory reaction was noted at the control sites treated with ointment base, as well as at untreated test sites [175]. Thus, since glucocorticoids suppress the inflammatory response to infection, this may be misinterpreted as a cure, even though the infection is still present. For this reason, too, the application of glucocorticoids to infectious skin changes is considered to be contraindicated, unless a reliably effective antimicrobial (broad-spectrum antimicrobial) is used in conjunction with the glucocorticoids.

Considering the diversity of skin changes associated with microbial invasion, it is understandable why antimicrobials are combined with glucocorticoids so frequently: Antimicrobials protect against the adverse effects of glucocorticoids. The clinical aspects of their combined use are discussed in Sect. 13.

Econazole nitrate is used together with triamcinolone acetonide in local therapy. Antagonistic interactions are avoided by administering these substances in a concentration ratio of 10:1 (1% and 0.1%). Miconazole (2%) is used together with hydrocortisone (1%) or depersolone (0.25%). Clotrimazole is under trial in an external preparation together with azidoamphenicol and dexamethasone. Isoconazole nitrate will be used together with diflucortolone valerate or flucortine butyrate [306a].

9 Microbial Infections in Man

9.1 General

"Microbial infections" is the term given to infections caused by bacteria and/or fungi. Microbial infections may be limited to body surfaces (skin and mucous membranes) or may invade deeper tissues.

An important factor in the occurrence of any infection is the disposition of the host (conditions of defense). This applies to superficial infections as well. The occurrence of infections also depends upon the type, virulence, and number of invading microorganisms.

Depending on the type of interaction between the microorganisms and the host, a distinction is made between parasitic infections which trigger a highly inflammatory defense reaction, and saprophytic infections which elicit no reaction from the host. Intermediate between these are "infections" by "facultatively-pathogenic organisms", which are limited to body surfaces. As a rule, these facultatively pathogenic organisms are saprophytes that proliferate to such a high degree ("colonization") that they can retard the healing of lesions. By definition, saprophytes live on dead matter; however, the metabolic products of such saprophytes can lead to toxic or allergic inflammations.

In infections of body surfaces, it is often a difficult task to distinguish between *primary* and *secondary* infections. Of course, classical pictures such as impetigo can be readily differentiated from a secondary "colonization" of inflammatory or degenerative skin lesions by staphylococci. But it is difficult to decide whether antimicrobial therapy is warranted for a "colonization," that is, for an overgrowth of essentially nonpathogenic saprophytes in lesions. Antimicrobial therapy should be instituted in case of doubt, however. Under practical therapeutic conditions, it is seldom possible to perform the recommended microbe count in order to differentiate between infected eczema and colonized (secondarily infected) eczema [166].

In fungal infections, too, a distinction is made between parasitic diseases and saprophytic mycoses. Between these extremes are the so-called "opportunistic mycoses", which are due more to factors on the part of the host than on the part of the fungi themselves. Dermatophytes are practically always the causative agents of true infections of the body surface. Yeasts and molds, on the other hand, are usually responsible only for secondary infections of preexisting skin lesions. The various types of lesion which are disposed to such opportunistic mycoses are discussed in Sect. 10.

In Europe, systemic fungus infections almost always take the form of opportunistic mycoses. Tropical regions are more favorable for the development of true systemic mycoses ("tropical mycoses").

Purely saprophytic diseases of the skin caused by bacteria or fungi include erythrasma, caused by a *Corynebacterium,* and pityriasis versicolor, caused by *Pityrosporum furfur.* The microbes blanket uninflamed skin areas like a lawn. The host manifests no defensive reaction. However, the organisms produce toxins which can impair pigment formation, for example.

Saprophytes on inflamed skin lesions (e. g., lesions due to contact eczema) must be evaluated differently from saprophytes on healthy skin. Even if the organisms were not the cause of the primary inflammation (as in impetigo), they can perpetuate the inflammation (retard healing) and even lead to infections of other individuals [166]. In such cases, an indication is present for antimicrobial therapy. On the other hand, the human skin surface is rich in saprophytes (see below) which represent an important part of the natural defenses against infection. It is often extremely difficult to correctly evaluate infections and colonizations and to come to a decision on the need for antimicrobial treatment, all from a clinical perspective.

9.2 Increase in Microbial Infections of Body Surfaces

An increase in microbial infections is reported in all branches of the medical profession. This is particularly true for superficial infections of the skin and mucous membranes.

Among the true infections, which must not be confused with secondary infections [232], the fungal diseases are the most significant. The increase in mycotic infections has been associated with numerous factors (see Sect. 10.2.). Some of these same factors are also responsible for the increase in bacterial infections. Primary bacterial infections of the skin or mucous membranes, and thus pyodermas in the strictest sense, are treated in most cases in the same way as infections of internal organs. Local measures generally are inadequate.

Secondary bacterial infections of inflamed skin lesions are difficult to evaluate. They may be true infections caused by pathogenic organisms, or may be due to an overgrowth of skin saprophytes. The uncertainty with respect to pathogenicity is reflected in the term "facultatively pathogenic organism."

The true skin-surface saprophytes have been the object of intensive study in recent years. From 40% to 80% of the staphylococci exhibit "antibiotic" activity; that is, they suppress the growth of pathogenic microorganisms. In one surgical department, for example, a strain of staphylococci resistant to the principal antibiotics proved highly sensitive to the metabolic products of a skin saprophyte [177, 286].

The skin-surface saprophytes include staphylococci *(Staph. aureus, Staph. albus)*, β-hemolytic streptococci (demonstrable on the skin of every fifth child, for example), diphtheroid rods and, in deeper strata, micrococci and lactobacilli [49, 123, 125, 194, 286].

Gram-negative organisms are of only minor importance as skin-surface saprophytes [125, 174]. They require considerably more moisture than gram-positive bacteria. As a result, gram-negative airborne microorganisms which reach the skin surface can survive there only a short time, at least at our latitudes. Gram-negative bacteria are also inhibited by an acidic medium. The normal pH of the skin surface largely prevents the survival of gram-negative rods. However, these organisms can thrive on the skin if sufficient moisture is present, as during heavy sweating. This has been confirmed in the tropics [174]. Gram-negative rods are present in intertriginous regions in almost half of all persons, though in relatively small numbers. A disturbance of the gram-positive organisms (antimicrobial deodorants) promotes the multiplication of gram-negative organisms.

Gram-negative organisms also appear whenever skin moisture is increased by inflammation (eczema) [297]. However, they are of no pathogenic importance; they disappear when the lesions heal. Some studies in humans showed that gram-negative organisms were present in a higher percentage of patients after the eruptions had healed than when the lesions were full-blown [122, 123]. Based on available observations, it must be concluded that gram-negative microorganisms are of little importance on the skin surface (cf. page 90).

The number of saprophytes which inhabit each square centimeter of skin surface depends upon the amount of moisture present, and thus upon individual factors. Moreover, the number of organisms will vary from site to site on the same individual. For example, 600 organisms/cm^2 may be present on the hip, 1900/cm^2 on the thigh, 30,000/cm^2 on the forehead, 1,350,000/cm^2 in the axilla and 7,600,000/cm^2 in the toewebs [175]. The total number of bacteria on the skin surface of a (clean) person is estimated at 11 billion.

The following conditions must be satisfied for a microbial infection of the skin surface to occur:
1) Invasion of pathogenic (or "facultatively" pathogenic) microorganism
2) Contamination by a large number of organisms
3) Adequate moisture
4) Damage to the skin
5) Overcoming of saprophytes
6) Overcoming of immune defense, the strength of which is the genetic factor determining whether infections occur easily or only in rare instances.

These conditions must also be satisfied when skin infections are induced experimentally [175].

If an *inflammatory* skin lesion harbors large numbers of bacteria (a limit of 10^6 organisms/cm^2 is assumed), these bacteria are of importance in the perpetuation of the lesion. Their metabolic products retard healing through toxic irritation, and sensitization to the chemical constituents or metabolic products of the bacteria is not uncommon [230, 333]. One of the main causes of the invasion of inflammatory lesions by microorganisms is increased moisture.

The microorganisms which can be detected in inflammatory skin lesions consist mostly of staphylococci *(Staphylococcus aureus)* [37, 122]. Yeasts are less commonly found [88]. Dermatophytes are practically never present as saprophytes [114].

One is struck by the absence of dermatophytes on the skin of persons suffering from atopic eczema. Ordinarily, dermatophyte infestation of the trunk can be demonstrated in about 4% of all persons living at our latitudes. The abnormal dryness of the skin of atopic patients does not create conditions favorable for dermatophytes. However, in very moist skin areas (in the toe-webs), the normal dermatophyte infestation (30%) is present even in atopic patients [99].

Sweat promotes fungal infections primarily by its moisture. The increase in amino acids on the skin surface of patients with tinea inguinalis and pityriasis versicolor is very probably due to an increased (infection-promoting) secretion of sweat. In patients with intertriginous candidosis, a smaller percentage content of squalene and bound carbohydrates has been demonstrated on healthy skin (as in diabetics). These shifts may well predispose the patient to candidoses and may also be associated with an increase in skin moisture [97].

With regard to the observed increase in infections, there is no sound evidence that a change in dispositional factors has taken place. Thus, this factor can hardly be held responsible for the increase in microbial infections of body surfaces. It is plain that our knowledge of skin and mucous membrane infections has grown, accompanied by continual improvements in diagnostic technique. But it is equally plain that the increase in microbial infections is *real*. This point will be discussed further in connection with mycotic infections in Sect. 10.2.

In conclusion, we must point out the great hygienic importance of the sometimes clinically inconspicuous superficial infection. Transmissions of infection have been repeatedly described [166]; those occurring in hospitals have even involved resistant strains of microorganisms, resulting, for example, in life-threatening complications in intensive care units. Such a danger is readily recognized in the case of microbial infections in the strict sense (furuncles, impetigo). However, in the case of inflammatory skin lesions harboring numerous microorganisms, it usually takes some time before these foci are identified as the source of transmissions.

9.3 Saprophytes and Parasites on Body Surfaces

The skin and mucous membrane surfaces are normally inhabited by bacteria. These bacteria, called saprophytes or commensals, are necessary for the maintenance of normal health (see above). Interestingly, far more anaerobic bacterial strains occur on the skin surface than aerobic strains. But the anaerobes are of no importance here [160] in contrast to the follicles in acne.

It cannot be stated that the saprophytes, the great majority of which are staphylococci, are absolutely nonpathogenic. Even saprophytes can exert adverse effects if stimulated (caused to multiply): enzyme release, toxin release, perhaps even allergen production. If certain saprophytes are stimulated, however, a disturbance of the skin-surface biology is already present. Saprophytes then become facultative pathogens, which can contribute to the pathogenesis of inflammatory dermatoses.

The staphylococci are the main etiologic agents of superficial skin infections (pathogenic microorganisms). But numerous other gram-positive bacterial strains also lead to superficial (as well as deep) infections of the skin and mucous membranes. By contrast, the gram-negative organisms are of only minor importance in *superficial* infections (for example cases cf. [305, 349]; gram-negative organisms occur as saprophytes on body surfaces only in exceptional circumstances (see above). They are most frequently encountered in the toewebs [193], where their pathogenic significance is unclear. However, the "gram negatives" are of considerable importance in systemic infections and *deeper* cutaneous infections (burns!).

Organisms of the genus *Pityrosporum* sometimes occur as saprophytic fungi on normal, healthy skin. These organisms become important pathogenically when overgrowth occurs, as may happen in acne vulgaris and seborrhea of the scalp. Inflammatory skin lesions are sometimes colonized by yeasts (usually of the genus *Candida*) (see Sect. 9.2). Dermatophytes, the classical etiologic agents of superficial mycoses, deep skin mycoses, and mycoses of the nail, are of no importance as secondary invaders of inflammatory lesions.

Experiments in laboratory animals have shown that the secondary infection of open wounds by yeasts is of importance. Yeasts interfere with wound healing, at least in rats [74].

When one considers the microflora in inflammatory skin and mucous membrane lesions, one must consider bacteria *and* fungi, although the bacteria play a much greater role according to previous results.

The anaerobes (bacterioids) present on all *mucous membranes* play a particularly important role. They can lead to severe (mostly opportunistic) infections if they spread to deeper tissues [160].

9.4 Mixed and Double Infections of Body Surfaces

The reasons for the presence of yeasts in bacterial infections and of bacteria in fungal infections are made clear by the results of basic *in vitro* research and animal experiments. Studies *in vitro* have demonstrated a mutual stimulation of metabolism between staphylococci *(Staphylococcus aureus)* and yeasts *(Can-*

dida albicans). The endotoxins of bacteria stimulate the growth (and pathogenicity?) of *Candida albicans* [68], while proteolytic products from *Candida albicans* serve as a substrate for the metabolism of *Staphylococcus aureus* [294].

Animal experiments have yielded similar results: If a mouse is injected intraperitoneally with suspensions of *Candida albicans*, staphylococci *(Staph. aureus)* can regularly be cultivated from the abscesses that form [295]. It has also been shown that *Staphylococcus aureus* promotes the transition of *Candida albicans* from the saprophytic to the parasitic stage [180].

These interactions, which permit bacteria and fungi to live in close association, can also be demonstrated on human skin: Staphylococci are commonly present in dermatophytic [149] and candidal [195] infections. On the other hand, fungi are not often found in bacterial skin infections, probably because the possibilities for fungal infections are more limited, and yeasts are not among the normal inhabitants of the human skin surface. Thus, primary mycotic infections can rapidly develop into double infections. The invading staphylococci can generally be assigned to the group of facultatively pathogenic organisms. If treatment of the fungal infection is effective, the staphylococci will disappear in most cases without specific treatment (return of the saprophytes). However, healing of the lesion can be hastened by treatment with drugs with both antifungal and antibacterial activity (e. g., the imidazole derivatives clotrimazole, miconazole, or econazole).

Mixed infections with different bacterial strains are relatively common, but infections with different strains of fungus are rare (e. g. [105]). This is also true of double infections [233]. An example of a *double fungal infection* would be intertriginous candidosis coexisting with interdigital dermatophytosis. Mixed infections with fungi and bacteria in the same lesion are not uncommon (see above).

10 Mycoses

10.1 Etiology of Mycoses

Parasitic mycoses are the result of infection by a large number of fungi (mycetes) that are pathogenic to man. In invasions by smaller numbers of fungi, the immune response and local defense (saprophytes) of the host will prevent the development of clinical symptoms, and no *mycosis* will occur.

Opportunistic mycoses develop only in the presence of certain factors on the part of the host (malnourishment, impaired defenses, congenital immune defects, immunosuppressive therapies). These host factors are more important for the development of an infection than factors on the part of the fungi themselves. At our latitudes the overwhelming majority of all systemic mycoses are of the opportunistic type. Systemic mycoses in children should raise the suspicion of a congenital immune defect syndrome [181]. It should be recalled that a certain toxin isolated from yeasts causes a disturbance of the immune response in laboratory animals. Yeast infections could develop via this route even if there were no primary injury to the host's defenses, and could thus "pave their own way" to a certain extent.

A host factor is also necessary in the case of superficial mycoses (exception: dermatophytoses). This factor may be a disturbance of the immune response, a metabolic disorder, or a local, preexisting lesion (sweat maceration, detergent damage, subacute and chronic eczemas). Diseases of the nails caused by yeasts and molds are almost always based on underlying circulatory or metabolic disturbances.

Humans can also contract a purely saprophytic mycosis in which the organisms blanket the skin like a dense lawn, without causing inflammation (Fig. 30). The disease is called *pityriasis versicolor.* The attendant disturbance of pigmentation is probably due less to the obstruction of light by the fungus lawn than to a toxic disturbance of pigment formation. The growth forms of the causative organism, *Pityrosporum furfur,* in culture are shown in Fig. 31.

Erythrasmas are *bacterial* saprophytic diseases affecting such areas as the inner thighs and axilla. These diseases spread only in very moist skin areas (intertriginous regions). In pityriasis versicolor, large portions of the trunk are affected.

Dermatophytoses are transmitted to man from other persons or from animals, either directly or via dead matter. Yeast and mold infections do not involve transmission in the true sense; the organisms are widespread, and factors on the part of the host are of critical importance in the occurrence of infections.

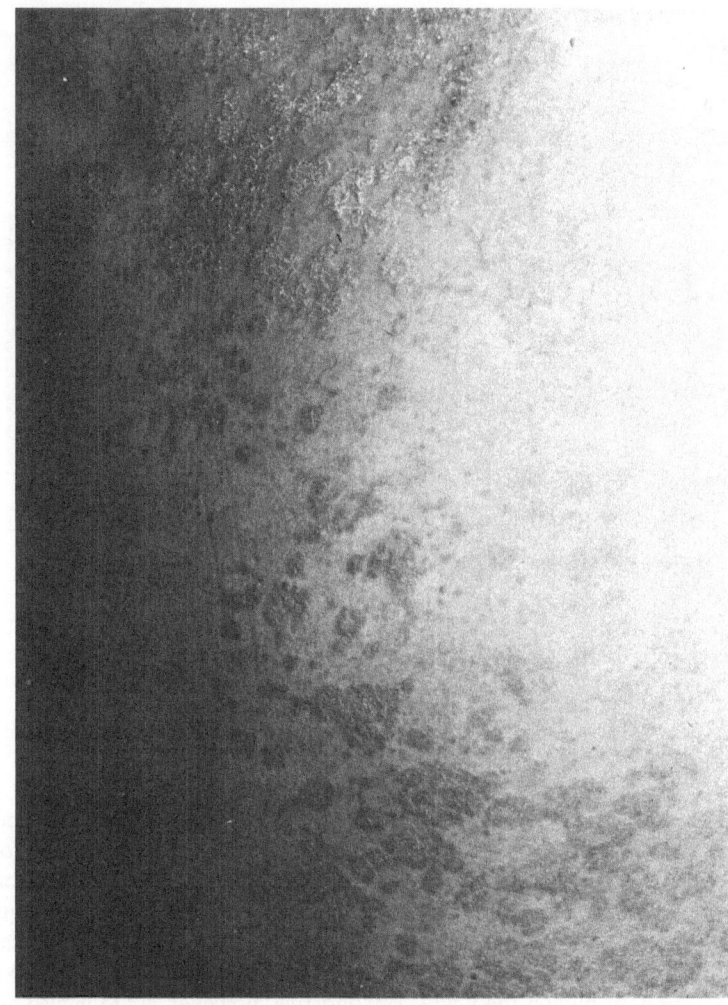

Fig. 30a. *Pityriasis versicolor.* Marked scaling is evident

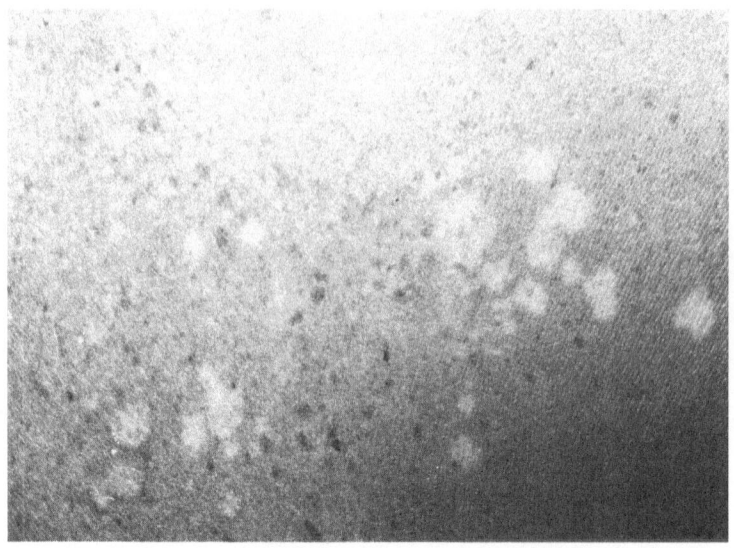

Fig. 30 b. No scaling, but marked changes in pigmentation

10.2 The Increase in Mycoses

10.2.1 General

A marked increase in mycoses has been observed in all branches of medicine during the last decade. Moreover, physicians have learned to look for mycoses even in cases that previously would not have raised suspicions of a fungal presence. This applies in particular to diseases caused by yeasts and molds, i. e., to the opportunistic mycoses. Greater experience with mycotic illnesses and the intensified search for fungi have undoubtedly contributed in part to the rise of mycoses in human medicine. Beyond this, however, there is also an absolute increase in mycotic infections, whose causes will be explored in this section.

Superficial infections with *dermatophytes* have already assumed epidemic proportions. Figures vary as to the scale of the epidemic. For example, a 10% incidence of mycosis was found during complete physical examinations of 22,000 persons at a large German hospital [183]. Dermatologic clinics report an incidence of 30%–40% for adults, 20% for juveniles, and up to 100% for swimmers [99, 255, 256, 306].

Even more pronounced is the increase in *opportunistic fungal infections*. Large surveys of many thousands of patients in the early 1960s indicated that the ratio of dermatophytoses to opportunistic fungal infections was 51% to 49% at that time. Today, surveys in comparable populations indicate a ratio of 32% to 68% (see [233]), even though the absolute number of dermatophytoses

94

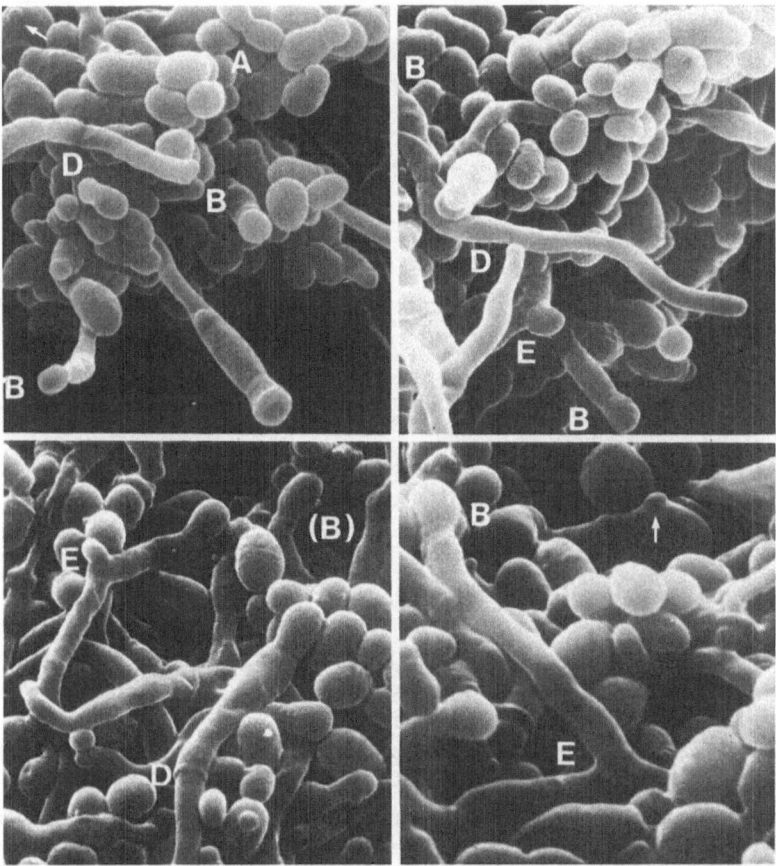

Fig. 31. *Scanning photomicrograph of Pityrosporum furfur in culture.* Various growth forms are seen: ovoid yeast cells (A) with budding (↗), spore formation from hyphae at the free ends (B), filamentation in hyphae (D) and mycelia with branchings (E, very rare). The growth of hyphae from yeast cells in the form of budding tubes is not shown here (after [47])

has markedly increased. Autopsies performed in the first decades of this century revealed opportunistic mycoses in less than 0.5%; in the same clinical center, mycoses were diagnosed in 0.3 to 1.3% in the years 1940 to 1970; since 1970, this percentage has increased up to 3.1% [141 a]. In patients with malignant cancer who had received immunosuppressive medication and/or radiation therapy, autopsies showed opportunistic fungal infections in 90% of the cases. The causative organisms in 80% of these cases were yeasts of the genus *Candida* [233].

In the field of *gynecology,* the ratio of trichomonas to candidal vaginitis was 5 : 1 at one time. Today this ratio is reversed [190], despite an absolute increase in trichomonas infections.

The increase in mycoses makes it necessary for physicians from all branches of medicine to take an interest in fungi, mycotic infections, and antimycotic therapies. Researchers, meanwhile, have been pressed to search for ever newer and better antimycotic drugs. This search has found a temporary conclusion in the family of imidazole derivatives. In terms of efficacy and tolerance, the imidazole derivatives are suited for use in all branches of medicine.

10.2.2 Increase in Mycoses Due to Medications

Although the factors responsible for the increase in mycoses cannot now be listed in order of importance, it is evident that *iatrogenic factors* must be considered as important, especially where *serious* infections are concerned.

Three groups of medications (and measures by the physician) promote the development of mycoses in man:
1) Immunosuppressive measures (immunosuppressive medications such as glucocorticoids and cytostatics, irradiation)
2) Antimicrobials
3) Hormones

Immunosuppression leads in a classical manner to opportunistic mycoses, caused mainly by yeasts and molds. The frequency with which opportunistic mycoses develop in patients treated for malignancies was mentioned above. In patients given cytostatics following organ transplantations (kidney transplants), there is an extremely high risk of fungal infection.

It is often recommended that prophylactic antimycotics be administered concurrently with immunosuppressive measures. With the imidazole derivatives now available, this recommendation can be safely followed. For completeness, it should be mentioned that fungal infections in tumor patients are not promoted by immunosuppressive measures alone. The immune response of most tumor patients is already impaired from the outset, and this undoubtedly contributes to their heightened susceptibility to opportunistic mycoses.

Antimicrobials can promote fungal infections by three mechanisms:
1) By the *selective destruction* of certain microorganisms, "vacancies" are created which can then be occupied by fungi (proliferation *in vacuo*). This mechanism is encountered with both antibacterial and antifungal agents, or after the administration of trichomonacidal drugs.
2) *Many antibiotics,* such as streptomycin, penicillin, or tetracycline, directly *stimulate the metabolism of yeasts and molds.* Tuberculostatic therapy occasionally gives rise to opportunistic mycoses which may lead to fatal complications in some circumstances (e. g., erosion of a pulmonary artery by a candidal infiltrate [229]). For further data see [352].
3) Yeasts and molds can also be *stimulated by products released by the decomposition of bacteria* (see also Sect. 9.4). Antibacterial substances cause bacteria to decompose; the products which are liberated by this process (endotoxins) promote the growth and stimulate the pathogenicity of yeasts.

The principal *hormones* to be considered besides the glucocorticoids (immunosuppression, see above) are the female *sex hormones,* which may provoke fungal infections (mainly vaginal candidosis). The taking of oral contraceptives leads to biochemical changes in the vaginal epithelium that resemble those occurring in pregnancy [208]. The increase in the glucose content and the pH shift from 3.0–4.5 to 5.5–6.5 promote the multiplication of yeasts, which are nearly always present, and a "levurosis," or yeast infection, may occur. In women taking oral contraceptives, the incidence of candidal vaginitis is just as high as in pregnant women during the first trimester (see p. 112): 10%–15%. It must be mentioned that figures up to 30% have also been reported.

The iatrogenic causes of opportunistic mycoses include various *measures by the physician,* whereby microorganisms are introduced into the body by way of various devices (catheters, dialyzers, respirators, heart-lung machines). Such devices cannot always be thoroughly sterilized. The risk of opportunistic fungal infections is especially great during intensive care, and in dialysis and transplant centers. The patient's natural defenses are lowered, and he is subjected to numerous procedures. Infection from infusion solutions is also possible. If unexplained fever develops in patients on antibacterial broad-spectrum antibiotics, with indwelling catheters, on high-caloric parenteral nutrition or under immunosuppressive therapy, candidosis must always be suspected [211].

Too little attention is given the fact that the organisms of opportunistic mycoses can also be spread through the repeated use of eye drops, ear drops, and perhaps even ointments.

10.2.3 Increase in Mycoses Due to Changes in Hygienic Habits and Modes of Social Behavior

Changes in vacationing habits (vacations on farms, trips abroad) and the increasing popularity of household pets (dogs, guinea pigs) are contributing to the rise of dermatomycoses in man. The more frequent use of such facilities as saunas, swimming pools, gymnasiums, and health spas is also increasing the possibilities of transmission.

Fungal infections in the region of the female genitalia are often attributable to an improper choice of clothing. For example, impermeable underclothing (synthetic fibers) or tight, poorly fitting pants promote infection by candidal organisms. Yeast fungi can practically always be found in *small numbers* in the female genital region. If an additional factor is added, such as the impermeable conditions and constant irritation produced by tight-fitting jeans, the fungi will be stimulated, and an infection will develop. The long-presumed connection between the use of feminine deodorant sprays and the occurrence of microbial infections has not been confirmed. The use of sprays containing antimicrobial agents (hexachlorophene) causes no significant disturbance of the microorganisms in the vulva and vagina [197]. Women who use vaginal sprays are usually sexually active; many also take oral contraceptives. The latter have created the erroneous impression that feminine deodorant sprays promote infections.

The increasing promiscuity and permissiveness of large segments of the population is another important factor contributing to the frequency of mycoses in the genital region, especially among women. According to the guidelines of the World Health Organization, candidosis of the external genitalia should be regarded as a sexually transmitted disease.

10.2.4 Increase in Mycoses Due to Metabolic Disturbances

The prosperity enjoyed in many countries has resulted in an increase in metabolic diseases. *Obesity* in itself promotes the development of opportunistic mycoses, for yeasts and molds thrive in the large, moist intertriginous areas characteristic of obesity (beneath the breasts, below the fat roll, in the groin area).

In *diabetes mellitus,* a capillaropathy is present which lowers the body's resistance to fungi. In *cardiovascular diseases* the supply of blood to the periphery is frequently diminished; this promotes fungal infections. Trophic disturbances of the nails (toenails) also invite invasion by fungi.

Metabolic disturbances which lead to severe itching, such as *cholestatic jaundice,* are usually accompanied by an increased incidence of microbial infections brought on by constant scratching.

Congenital and acquired immune defects, leukemias, diseases of the reticuloendothelial system, etc. promote the occurrence of opportunistic fungal diseases by depressing the body's natural defenses (see pg. 88).

10.2.5 Increase in Mycoses Due to Physical Influences

The increasing exposure of our bodies to injurious physical influences of various kinds could perhaps contribute to the increased incidence of mycoses. On the one hand, physical influences can lead to skin damage that creates a portal of entry for pathogenic fungi (e. g., radiation damage to the finger of a radiologist [100]). On the other hand, certain physical influences are capable of activating fungi. Exposure to ultrasound (in higher-than-therapeutic intensities) causes a marked acceleration of growth in *Scopulariopsis brevicaulis* [29]. No studies are yet available on the effects of lower intensities.

10.3 Classification of Mycoses

Mycoses are diseases which are caused by fungi. Fungi are eukaryotic thallophytes belonging to the plant kindgom. They lack chlorophyll and so are incapable of photosynthesis. The various types of fungi are classified according to the D-Y-M system (dermatophytes, yeasts, molds) as regards their relevance to human medicine.

Dermatophytes cause infections of the skin, hair, and nails. The skin infections may be superficial (tinea superficialis) or deep (tinea profunda) (Figs. 32 and 33). The internal organs are not affected.

Yeasts and molds cause practically only opportunistic mycoses at our latitudes. The infections may consist of superficial or deep (granulomatous) skin and mucous membrane changes that may become generalized and involve the internal organs.

Systemic mycoses are fungal infections of various internal organs. At one time systemic mycoses were limited to countries outside Europe (see Sect. 10.6), hence the term "tropical mycoses." But increased travel abroad and especially disturbances of the immune system during modern chemotherapy for malignancies have led to a rising incidence of systemic yeast and mold infections in Central Europe as well.

10.4 Mycoses of the Skin and Mucous Membranes

10.4.1 General

Dermatomycoses is the term given to infections with various dermatophytes. The different forms of tinea are encountered in numerous areas of the body (tinea inguinalis, tinea pedis, tinea manuum, tinea capitis, etc.).

It is not necessary here to discuss the individual dermatophytes (strains of *Trichophyton* and *Microsporum*) and forms of tinea. But certain important facts should be mentioned. Dermatomycoses in Central Europe are most frequently caused by *Trichophyton rubrum* and *Trichophyton mentagrophytes* (identified by form and color in culture; cannot be identified by direct examination of clinical specimens). Only 5% of dermatophytoses are pure epidermophytoses (causative organism: *Epidermophyton floccosum,* a strain of dermatophyte that attacks only the epidermis, but not the hair).

Tinea nigra, a superficial dermatomycosis caused by *Cladosporium wernecki* and marked by dark brown to black spots on the palms of the hands (Fig. 34), is native to the tropics but is sometimes brought to Europe by travelers. Diseases occurring exclusively in the tropics are tokelau (tinea imbricata), caused by *Trichophyton concentricum,* and tinea oceanica, caused by *Trichophyton oceanicum* (Figs. 35 and 36).

The danger of *tinea pedis* (Fig. 37), the trivial fungal infection of the foot, lies in its ability to act as a portal of entry for bacterial infections, such as erysipelas. Trivial mycoses of the feet can also cause tinea profunda granulomatosa of the lower leg, especially in women. Areas which are rubbed by synthetic-fiber stockings and the hard matting agents (titanium dioxide) con-

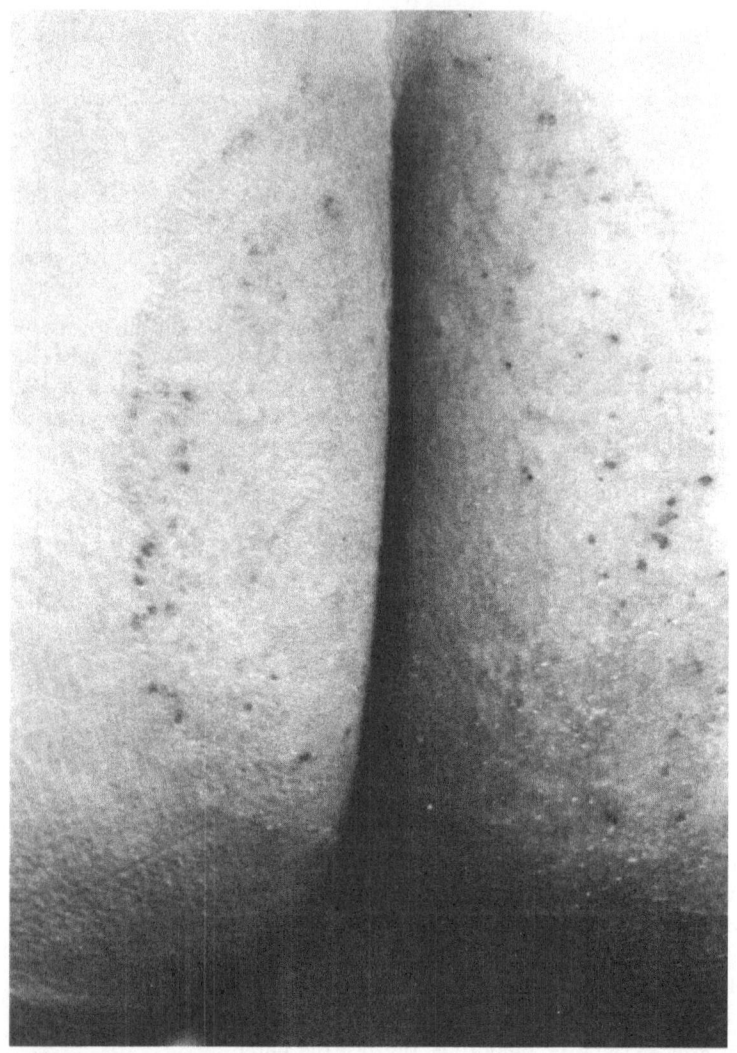

a

Fig. 32 a–d. *Tinea superficialis.* Tinea glutaealis (**a**), tinea corporis on the neck (**b**), on the forearm (**c**) and on skin of a Negro (**d**)

tained in them may become infected with dermatophytes, followed by the development of deep-seated nodules.

The danger of *tinea manuum* (Fig. 38), the trivial fungus disease of the hand, is its ability to serve as a portal of entry for sensitizations. For this reason, mycoses of the hand are of great importance in occupational medicine. There is a need for rapid and effective treatment, even if only discrete changes are present [232]. Mycoses of the skin between the toes may be caused by derma-

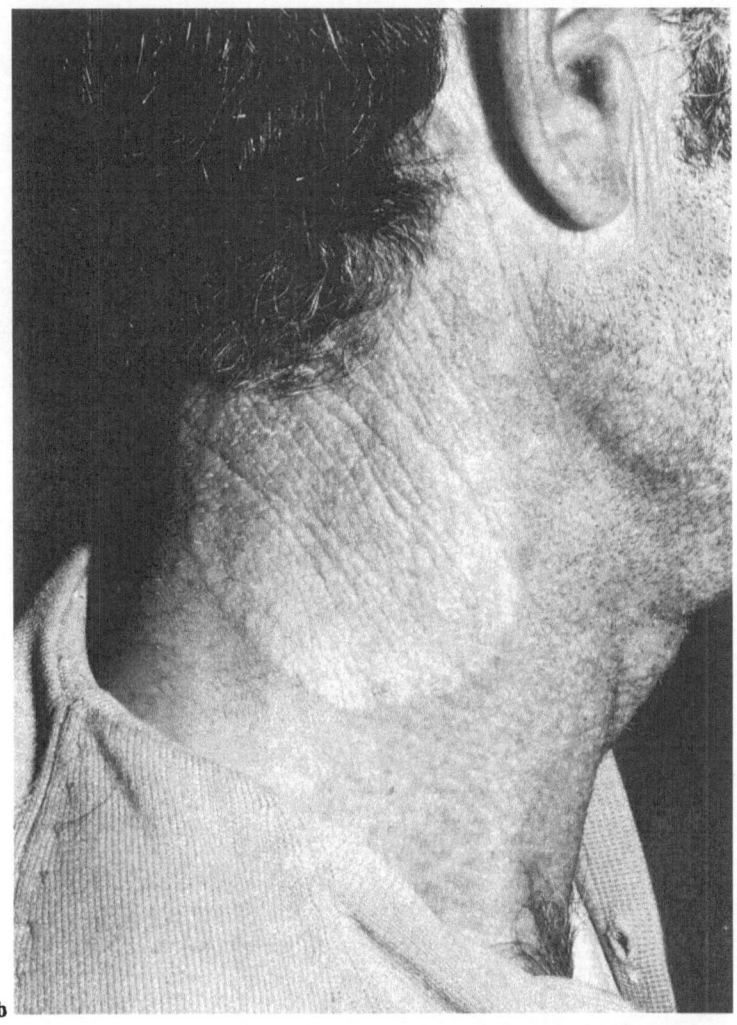

b

tophytes (37%), yeasts (60%), or molds (3%). These diseases are best treated with substances that are active against all three groups of fungi, such as the imidazole derivatives.

Opportunistic mycoses of the skin exist in many forms. Mixed infections with staphylococci are the most common. The most frequent sites of infection are the intertriginous regions, the interdigital regions (see above), the corners of the mouth, and the nail bed. Occasionally yeasts can also be detected on eczematous skin lesions, where they cause the formation of vesicles and pustules. Mycoses of the mucous membranes are almost always opportunistic (e. g., vaginitis, otitis, stomatitis, proctitis). It remains uncertain whether my-

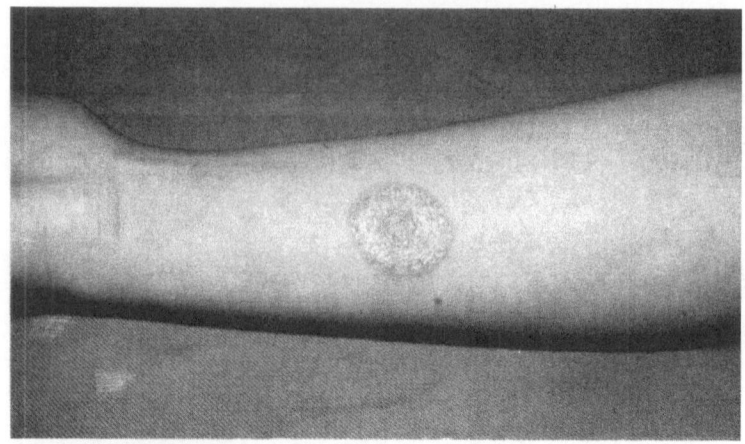

Fig. 32 c

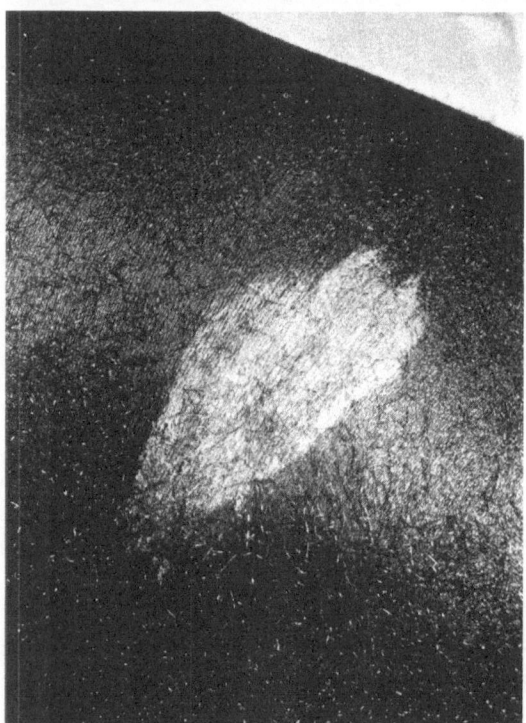

Fig. 32 d

cotic keratitis (keratomycosis) must be regarded as opportunistic in all cases, especially when the infection is caused by *Fusarium* or *Cephalosporium* species.

Candidoses, both systemic and local, are becoming increasingly important in man [198]. Affections of the skin include erosio interdigitalis candidamycetica, candidal intertrigo and candidal paronychia. The predisposing local factors

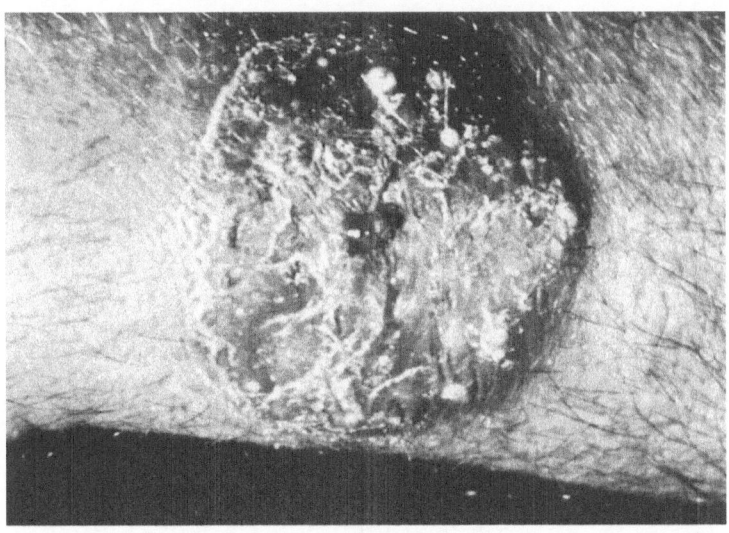

Fig. 33. *Tinea profunda corporis*

are a moist environment, disturbances of metabolism or blood flow and, in paronychia, frequent contact with carbohydrates (bakers, for example). Folliculitis and secondarily infected eczemas caused by *Candida* are less common.

The most common *mucosal candidosis* is vaginitis. This disease is marked by itching, with malodorous, yellow-white coatings on the mucous membranes and a caseous discharge. Erosions sometimes appear on the labia. If allowed to persist, the infection may lead to micturition difficulties and dyspareunia. The skin of the perigenital region is only rarely affected (folliculitis, vesicles, pustules). The anal region is involved in 50% of the cases; rectal candidosis may be present, too, and cause persistent recurrences, cf. [158]. Balanoposthitis frequently develops in the sexual partners of candidal vaginitis patients.

The second most common mucosal candidosis is stomatitis. From 30% to 70% of all denture wearers suffer from candidal stomatitis [233, 273, 291], which is marked by erythema, coatings (also on the denture) and papillary hyperplasia. Anguli infectiosi (perlèche) are often present as well. Other important mucosal infections caused by *Candida* are otitis media and sinusitis.

The importance of *Candida* in perioral dermatitis is unclear. Many case reports indicate complete healing under antimycotic therapy (see [45], for example). The fact of positive intracutaneous reactions proves nothing, because similar test results can also be obtained in healthy persons. The observation of *Candida* is of no importance in acne vulgaris. Mixed infections with bacteria and *Candida albicans* are often present on chronically steroid-damaged skin, which is sometimes the basis for perioral dermatitis (see Sect. 9).

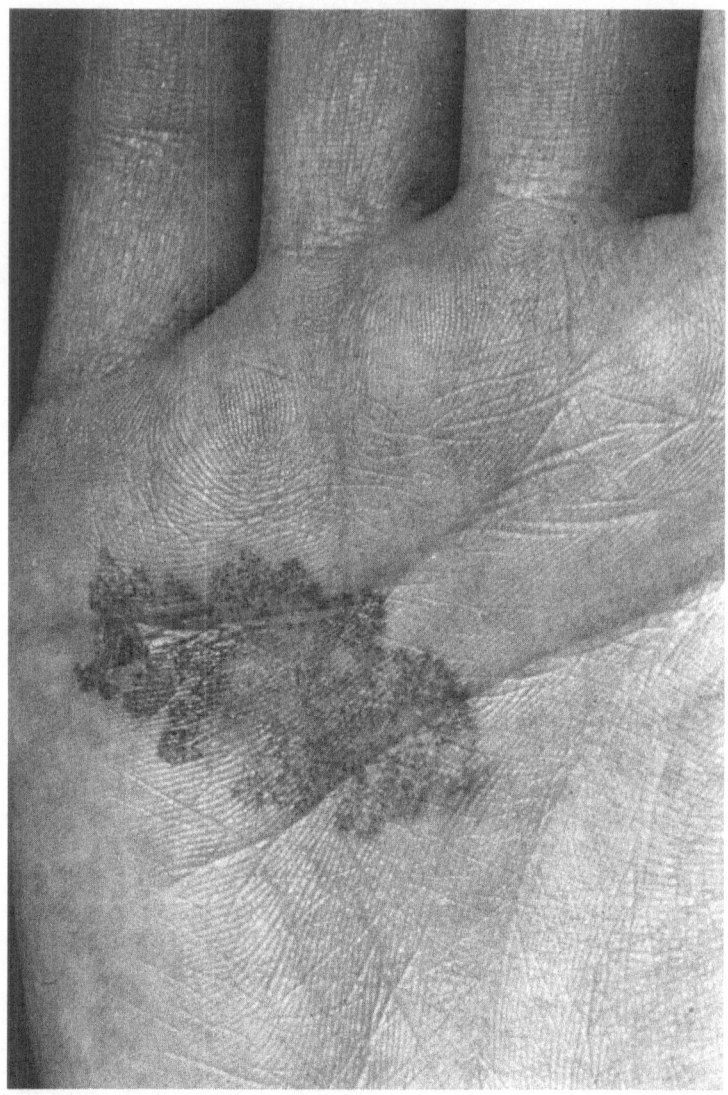

Fig. 34. *Tinea nigra.* An increasing incidence of this infection is observed in Europe (infection is carried in by travelers; it is nontransmissible in Europe)

Chronic, mucocutaneous candidoses are the result of severe disturbances of the cellular immune response (e. g., familial immune defect syndrome); for review, cf. [182]. Antibodies against candidal cell-wall antigens are found in the serum of all candidosis patients; antibodies against cell-content antigens are found only in patients with systemic candidoses. The number of allergies to molds is surprisingly high [4, 256].

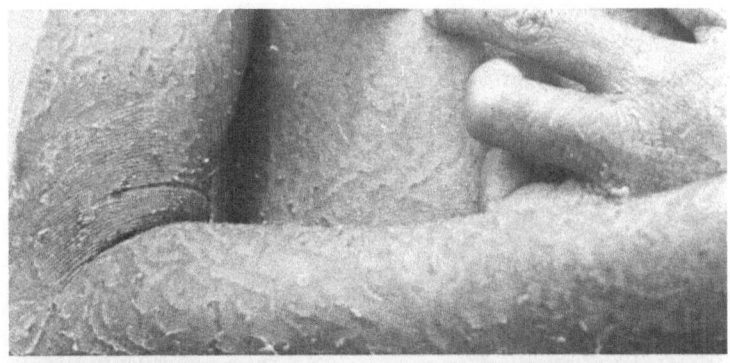

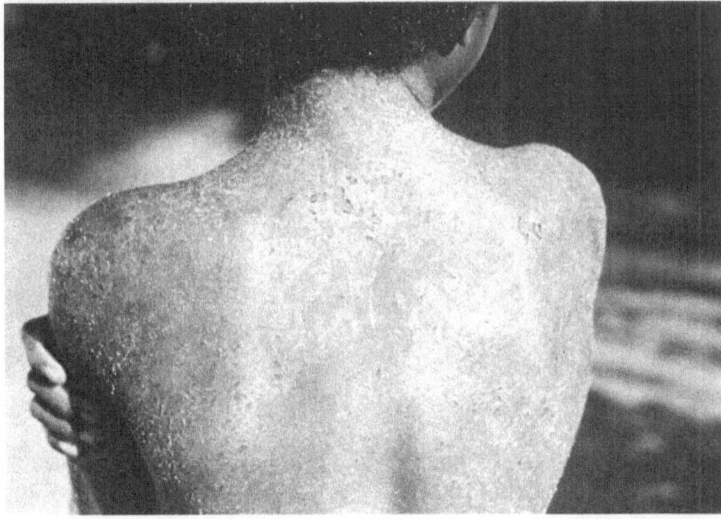

Fig. 35. *Superficial mycosis of tropical regions:* Tokelau. Anterior view *(top)* and posterior view *(bottom)*

10.4.2 Diagnosis of Skin and Mucous Membrane Mycoses

Superficial mycoses are diagnosed:
1) From the clinical picture (cf. [61])
2) By the direct examination of clinical specimens
3) By demonstrating the organism in culture (only means of exact *identification* of the causative organism)

Deep (systemic) mycoses are diagnosed:
1) From the clinical picture
2) By demonstrating the organism in culture
3) By detecting changes in the immune status (skin tests, serologic antibody tests)

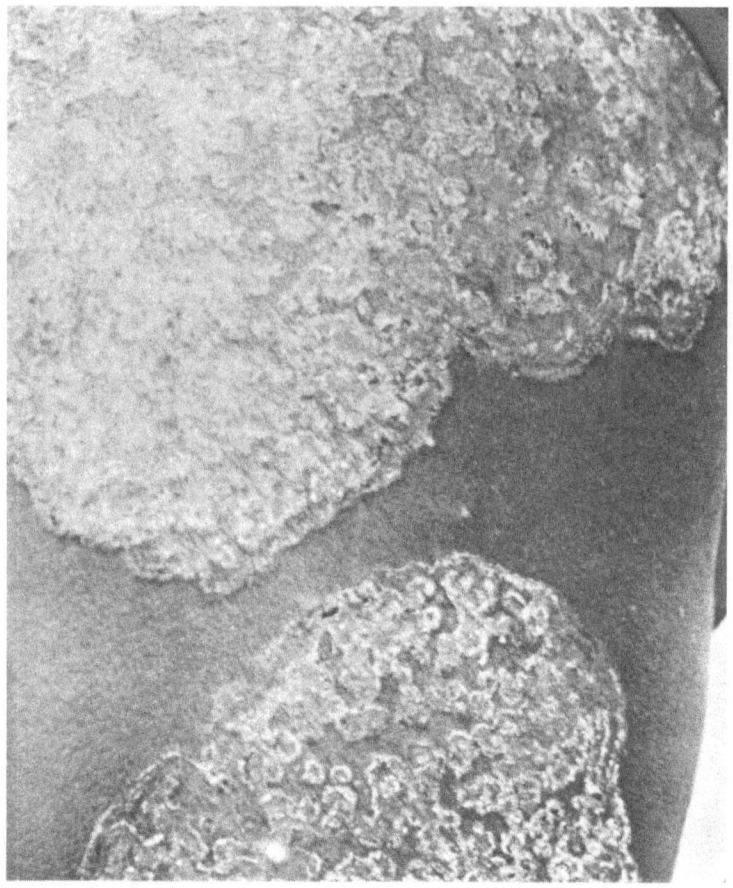

Fig. 36. *Tinea superficialis oceanica* caused by *Trichophyton oceanicum*

Mycoses of the female genitalia are diagnosed:
1) From the clinical picture
2) By the direct examination of clinical specimens

A positive fungus culture demonstrates only the presence of fungi. Under some circumstances (e. g., a low count) these fungi cannot be regarded as the causative organisms of the infection.

A *cure is demonstrated* by the assessment of clinical symptoms (clinical cure) and by the absence of fungal growth in culture. Fungus elements seen in clinical specimens may be due to dead organisms.

In practice, superficial mycoses are diagnosed by the direct examination of clinical preparations. The clinical specimen is treated with 20% potassium hydroxide solution, is heated and, after cooling, is examined under the microscope with low illumination. Fungus elements are visible as double-contoured,

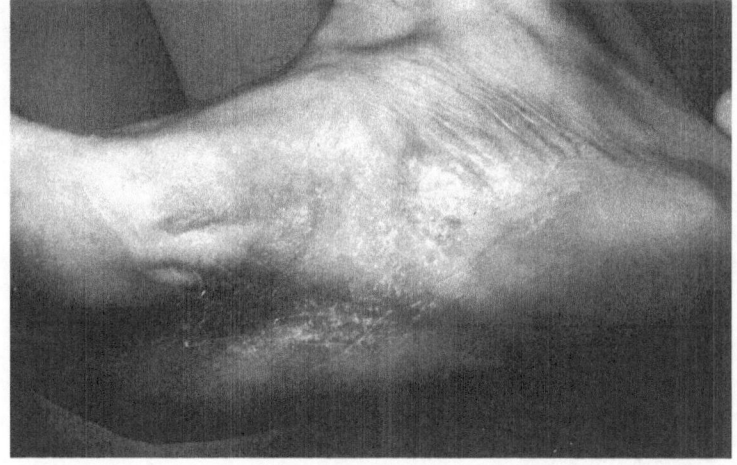

a

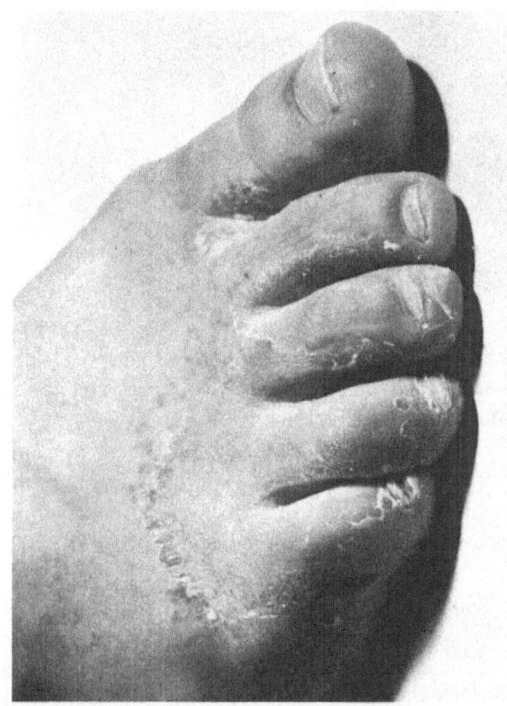

b

Fig. 37 a–c. *Mycoses of the feet.* Dermatophyte infection of the arch of the foot (**a**) and interdigital dermatophytosis (**b**). The changes on the underside of the toes and between the toes (**c**) may be caused by dermatophytes or may be due to the invasion of sweat-macerated skin by yeasts or bacteria

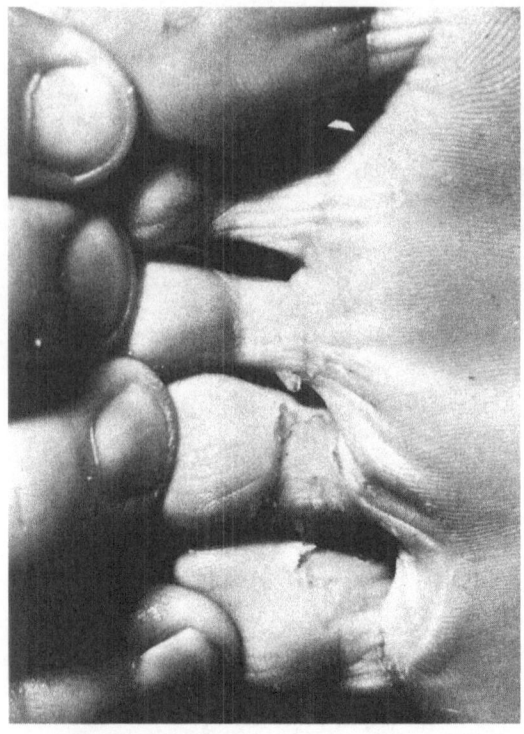

Fig. 37c

branched, septate filaments, or as ovules. When Parker's ink is added to the potassium hydroxide, these structures are not stained and therefore stand out sharply against the dark background.

It is not possible to distinguish between dermatophytes and yeasts by direct examination. Yeasts *(Candida albicans)* exhibit a dimorphism: Budding cells (ovules) are present in saprophytic stages, while pseudomycelia are formed in parasitic stages. This may cause them to be mistaken for dermatophytes; examples are shown in Figs. 39 and 40 [256].

Cultivation is resorted to only in relatively rare cases. It is not always possible and is worth the considerable effort only in certain cases, as for example to determine whether mycotic nail infections in older patients are caused by dermatophytes (indication for long-term oral griseofulvin therapy). If trophic disturbances of the nail are present, it is entirely possible that the mycosis is opportunistic, and griseofulvin therapy would be useless. In younger patients with no signs of any infection-promoting disorders, pathogen identification is more easily dispensed with at the start of griseofulvin therapy.

Unfortunately, combined infections with dermatophytes and *Scopulariopsis* (which is insensitive to griseofulvin) frequently occur. This poses special diagnostic and therapeutic problems (oral ketoconazole!).

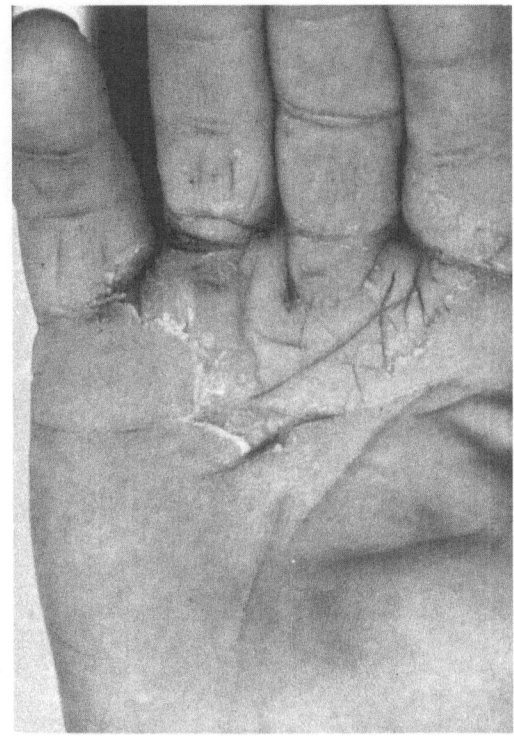

Fig. 38. *Tinea manuum*

In superficial mycoses, an adequate diagnosis can be made on the basis of the clinical picture and direct microscopic findings. Broad-spectrum antimycotics are just as effective in the presence of dermatophytes as in the presence of yeasts or molds. In this sense the imidazole derivatives have simplified the treatment of fungal infections and increased the likelihood of a cure.

10.5 Mycoses of the Female Genitalia

Vaginitis and vulvitis due to fungi are included among the opportunistic mycoses. The principal causative organisms are yeasts (*Candida* species). About 60% of all vaginitis cases are caused by yeasts, while about 20% are caused by trichomonads. The remaining 20% consist of "nonspecific" forms (traumatic irritations, bacteria). Vaginitis is best diagnosed by the examination of smears (see Sect. 10.4.1).

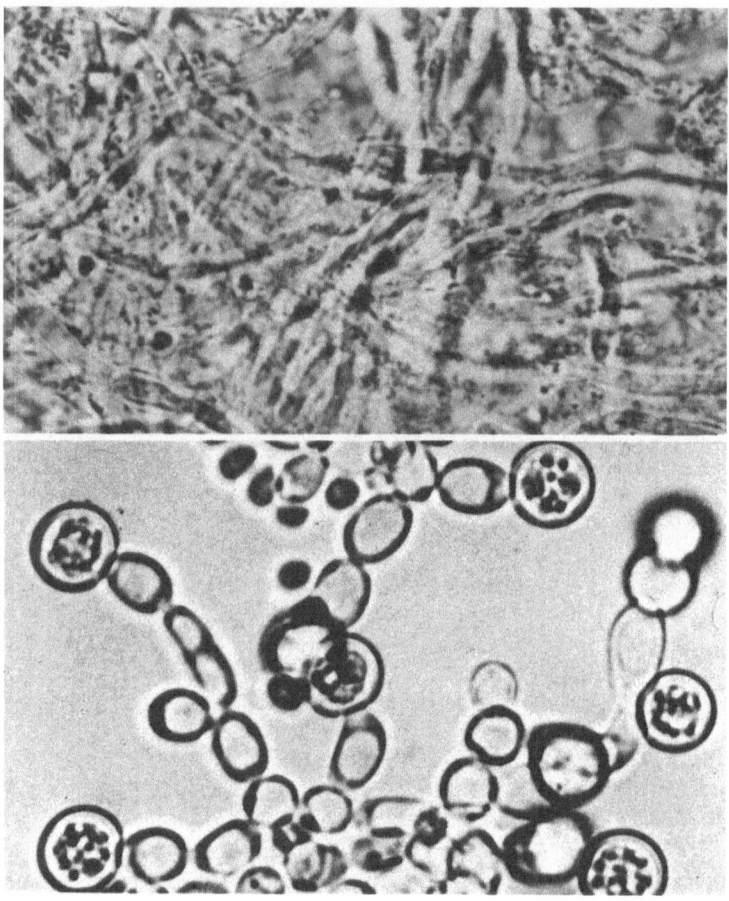

Fig. 39. *Candida albicans in the parasitic and saprophytic stage. Top:* Direct examination of nail plate. Only hyphae are visible; no budding cells are seen. *Bottom:* Culture on rice extract agar. Numerous chlamydospores and pseudomycelia are seen

Cultivation is meaningful only if corresponding clinical symptoms are present. Yeasts can often be demonstrated in the vaginal smears of healthy women as well. But these few fungi will give a positive result in culture. A positive culture on Nickerson's medium indicates only the presence of a *levurosis* (yeast fungus infection); it cannot disclose whether a candidosis or torulopsidosis is present. On the other hand, the number of yeasts can be assessed by examining stained vaginal smears. Cultivation is the best means of proving the efficacy of a therapeutic measure, for a negative culture is the most stringent criterion for the destruction of all fungi. However, a complete clinical cure is frequently reported despite still positive culture findings (see above).

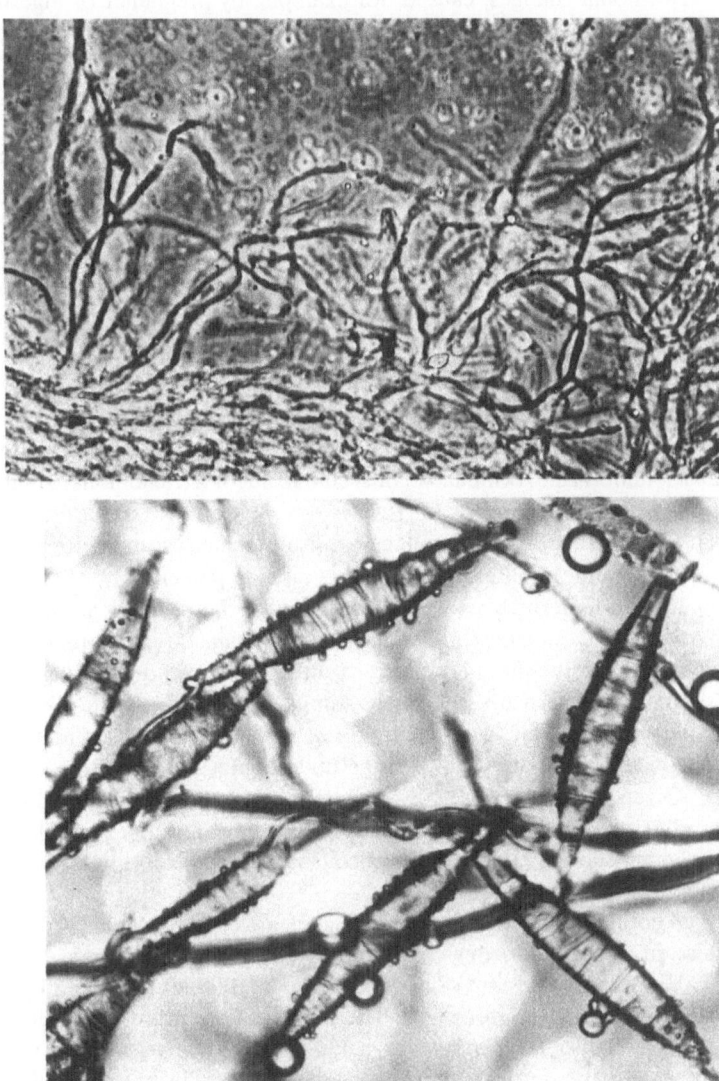

Fig. 40. *Dermatophytes in the parasitic and saprophytic stage. Top:* Direct examination of KOH mount of skin scrapings. Only hyphae are seen. *Bottom:* Culture on Kimmig agar. The typical rough-walled macroconidia are visible on the aerial mycelium *(Microsporum canis)*

It is well known that yeasts of the genus *Candida* essentially are endosaprophytes which normally are encountered in the human digestive tract or on the vulvovaginal mucosa. The transformation of these yeasts – the most important strain being *Candida albicans* – from the saprophytic state to the pathogenic "infectious" state may be conditioned by various factors:

Hormonal changes, caused, for example, by pregnancy or ingestion of oral contraceptives, leading to an increased glycogen content of the epithelial cells

Metabolic diseases (diabetes mellitus) and diseases of the immune system (leukemia, Hodgkin's disease)

Medications provoking a depression of the immune system (cytostatics, corticosteroids) or interfering with the microbial balance (broad-spectrum antibiotics)

Professions which necessitate a prolonged contact with water, carbohydrates, or macerating chemical substances. People at risk in this way include cannery workers, laundry workers, workers in fermentation industries (e. g., brewing), and bakers

A classic example of opportunistic mycosis is candidal vaginitis resulting from the systemic administration of antitrichomonal drugs. Candidal vaginitis is observed in about 20% of women treated orally with metronidazole, tinidazole, nimorazole, ornidazole, or secnidazole for a trichomonal infection. *There are three possible reasons for this:*

1) The destruction of anaerobic organisms creates vacancies for microbes. This leads to the proliferation of yeasts already present.
2) Imidazole derivatives with substituents at the nitrogen atom in the 5 position – and only these are effective orally against trichomonads – damage the vaginal epithelium and interfere with the natural defenses against yeasts.
3) Imidazole derivatives directly stimulate the growth and pathogenicity of yeasts. However, such an action has been ruled out for metronidazole in concentrations between 0.1 and 500 $\mu g/ml$ [250].

Given the frequency with which systemic antitrichomonal therapy leads to candidal vaginitis, local prophylaxis is now almost routinely employed, e. g., by the application of clotrimazole, miconazole, or econazole in the form of vaginal suppositories or cream [209].

Another example of opportunistic mycosis is the vaginal (and rectal) candidosis in women following X-ray therapy of genital carcinomas [113].

Vaginal mycoses are of importance to the patient herself and, during pregnancy, to the newborn as well. The *patient* suffers from the clinical symptoms (see Sect. 10.4.1). Of particular significance is the dyspareunia, which may be the most marked symptom in rare cases. This results in sexual difficulties, and alienation of the partners often occurs. Vaginal mycoses have frequently been cited as a cause of sterility.

The incidence of candidal vaginitis increases with the duration of pregnancy. The incidence is 10% during the first trimester, rising to 50% by the third trimester [81]. If vaginal candidosis is present at the time of delivery, there is a 40%–80% chance that the infection will be transmitted to the *newborn*. Sometimes the infection is asymptomatic, and *Candida* organisms may be carried into intensive care units by premature infants [278, 279]. Increasingly, antimycotic therapy is administered to *all pregnant women* 4 weeks before term as a precautionary measure.

Candidal vaginitis is almost always accompanied by candidal vulvitis. The anal region is involved in about half the patients. From 40% to 60% of the sexual partners of women with candidal vaginitis contract candidal balanitis (balanoposthitis).

Vaginitis caused by *Candida albicans* is present in about every second or third patient with vaginal mycosis. Other yeasts which are pathogenically important in vaginitis are *Candida tropicalis* and strains of *Rhodotorula*.

10.6 Systemic Mycoses

Systemic mycoses in the strict sense ("tropical" mycoses) consist of a group of six diseases: North American blastomycosis (caused by *Blastomyces dermatitidis*); paracoccidioidomycosis (= South American blastomycosis, caused by *Blastomyces brasiliensis*), and coccidioidomycosis (caused by *Coccidioides immitis*); cryptococcosis, formerly called torulosis (caused by *Cryptococcus neoformans*); sporotrichosis (caused by *Sporothrix schenkii*); histoplasmosis (caused by *Histoplasma capsulatum*); and chromomycosis (caused by *Hormodendrum compactum*).

Opportunistic systemic mycoses in cases of immune defects, chronic antibiotic therapy, cytostatic therapy, etc. are attributable to a large number of pathogens [28]. *Candida albicans* and strains of *Aspergillus* are the most common causative agents. Systemic mycoses require systemic treatment.

10.7 General Principles in the Treatment of Mycoses

10.7.1 Systemic Treatment

Various methods are available for the treatment of organic mycoses and deep cutaneous mycoses: The use of chemotherapeutic agents (imidazole derivatives, griseofulvin, amphotericin B-deoxycholate complex, 5-fluorocytosine), the administration of transfer factor (mixture of polypeptides and oligonucleotides, prepared from human lymphocytes; molecular weight about 10,000), and immune stimulation (vaccination, levamisole, see [238]).

The amphotericin B-deoxycholate complex can be administered intravenously, intrathecally (for meningitis), intraperitoneally (irrigation), and intraarticularly [43, 219, 202]. The toxicity of this soluble polyene complex is relatively high: In doses of 1 mg/kg body weight, amphotericin B causes reversible kidney damage (60% of patients), irreversible kidney damage (20% of patients), severe general reactions such as fever and spasms (50%-80% of patients), a fall of hemoglobin values (30%–50% of patients) and thrombophlebitis (20% of patients) [26]; the methyl ester is less toxic [347].

The antimicrobial activity of amphotericin B against the organisms of systemic mycoses is given in Table 17. The effectiveness of amphotericin B in the treatment of aspergillosis is unclear; in blastomycosis, coccidioidomycosis, candidosis, and histoplasmosis, amphotericin B gives good results in about 50% of the cases. Nevertheless, amphotericin B is still considered the drug of choice in the treatment of coccidioidomycosis, histoplasmosis, aspergillosis, and phycomycosis. It is recognized as a second-line drug for treatment of blastomycosis, candidosis, cryptococcosis, sporotrichosis, and (local) chromomycosis [26].

The drug *5-fluorocytosine* is an antimetabolite which is tolerated relatively well in daily doses of 100–200 mg/kg body weight. It is deaminated in the yeast cell to 5-fluorouracil, which is incorporated into ribonucleic acids instead of uracil. This renders the RNA incapable of protein synthesis. 5-Fluorocytosine may be administered orally. As for adverse effects, disturbances of liver function and hemopoiesis have been reported.

The spectrum of 5-fluorocytosine is shown in Table 17. The value of 5-fluorocytosine in systemic mycotic therapy is limited, for yeasts acquire a rapid mutative resistance (change in active transport mechanisms through the cell wall, change of deaminase activity in the cell plasma, inhibition of the phosphorylation of uracil or 5-fluorouracil for incorporation into RNA). Ten percent of the *Aspergillus* and *Candida* strains exhibit a *primary* resistance to the drug [214]. Consequently, 5-fluorocytosine may be administered only after the resistance of the pathogen has been determined. If an absence of resistance has been demonstrated, 5-fluorocytosine is the drug of choice in the treatment of candidosis, torulopsidosis, cryptococcosis and chromomycosis [26, 280].

Table 17. Minimum inhibitory concentrations of amphotericin B, 5-fluorocytosine and econazole for the organisms causing systemic mycoses

| Organism | Minimum inhibitory concentrations in µg/ml | | |
	Amphotericin B	5-Fluoro-cytosine	Econazole
Candida albicans	0.5	0.1–10	1.0
Aspergillus species	0.8	1.0–10	0.01
Torulopsis glabrata	0.5	0.1–10	0.1
Cryptococcus neoformans	0.2	0.5–15	0.1
Histoplasma capsulatum	1.0	> 500	0.01
Coccidioides immitis	2.0	> 500	[a]
Blastomyces dermatitidis	12.0	> 500	0.01
Hormodendrum compactum	15.0	–	[a]
Sporothrix schenckii	8.0	–	0.01

[a] No data available.

Amphotericin B and 5-fluorocytosine can also be combined for treatment of systemic mycoses in some circumstances (daily dose 0.3 mg/kg amphotericin B plus 100–150 mg/kg 5-fluorocytosine). Problems of pathogen resistance can be overcome in this way [280, 337].

The latest and probably the best group of systemic antimycotic agents are the *imidazole derivatives*. Initial clinical results indicate that the introduction of this group of drugs, especially of the newest compound ketoconazole (see Sect. 13), has significantly improved results in the systemic treatment of mycoses. Expectations must be lowered in cases of opportunistic systemic mycoses, however, because the underlying disturbance usually cannot be corrected.

The importance of *griseofulvin* is limited to dermatology. The introduction of griseofulvin into the systemic therapy of dermatophyte infections (superficial and deep tinea, onychomycoses) revolutionized the treatment of dermatomycoses. The oral administration of griseofulvin in microcrystalline form (particle size less than 2.6 μm) in a single daily dose of 500 mg is highly effective [98, 160]. Dermtophytoses, trichophytoses, and microsporoses are completely cured without relapse within a period of four weeks. For onychomycoses, treatment must be continued until the nail is completely renewed; if blood flow to the lower extremities is impaired, this may take up to two years.

Oral griseofulvin therapy should not be considered the first-line treatment for superficial dermatophytoses. Systemic medication is indicated only after all possibilities of local treatment have been exhausted. In onychopathy caused by griseofulvin-sensitive fungi, however, oral griseofulvin therapy should be instituted without delay.

10.7.2 Local Antimycotics

An almost limitless number of substances are already available for use in the local treatment of mycotic infections. Substances with good antifungal activity are found in all classes of antimicrobial drugs (antiseptics, chemotherapeutic agents, etc.). For reviews cf. [10, 160, 329].

The most important groups of local antimycotics are the following: Phenols and phenol derivatives, salicylic acid and halogenated salicylic acid derivatives, carboxylic acids, aromatic sulfides and sulfones, 8-hydroxyquinolines, triphenylmethane dyes, phosphonium and ammonium bases, organic mercury compounds, and thiocarbamates (tolnaftate). The most widely used antibiotics are the polyenes: nystatin, natamycin, amphotericin B, and variotin.

Practically all the substances and classes of substances mentioned have adverse effects. Some exhibit a very low antifungal activity in vivo, resulting in an absence of antimycotic (antimicrobial) activity in deeper skin layers (salicylic acid), while others lead to photosensitizing effects (halogenated organic compounds) or systemic toxic reactions at higher concentrations (hexachlorophene). Other substances, in turn, interfere with thyroid function tests performed during therapy (clioquinol), or cause irritation (quinoline derivatives), sensitization (quinoline derivatives, variotin), or discoloration (nystatin, amphotericin B, triphenylmethane dyes). Still other antimycotics are poorly tolerated by the mucous membranes (surface-active agents, quarternary bases) or have an insufficient activity spectrum (tolnaftate, pyrrolnitrin, nystatin). These questions have already been discussed in Sect. 2 and 8.

As knowledge has increased on the various types of fungi occurring on the skin and their importance in disease, interest has grown in the "broad-spectrum antimycotics," which exhibit strong activity against all fungi pathogenic to man. Combinations of dermatophyte-active substances (e. g., tolnaftate) and yeast-active antibiotics (e. g., nystatin) have not proved quite satisfactory.

Besides the imidazole derivatives, the following substances are now included in the arsenal of broad-spectrum antimycotics: *haloprogin* (2,4,5-trichloro-phenyl-iodopropargyl ether), *clioquinol* (5-chloro-7-iodo-8-hydroxyquinoline), *chlorquinaldol* (5,7-dichloro-2-methyl-8-hydroxyquinoline), *triclosan* (2,4,4'-trichloro-2'-hydroxydiphenyl ether) and ciclopirox. The structural formulas of these substances are shown in Fig. 41. The minimum inhibitory concentrations of certain broad-spectrum antimycotics are given in Table 18.

The data in the table are mean values. Because the inhibition tests were performed on various strains of microorganisms by various authors, the table provides only a general overview. Direct comparisons are not possible.

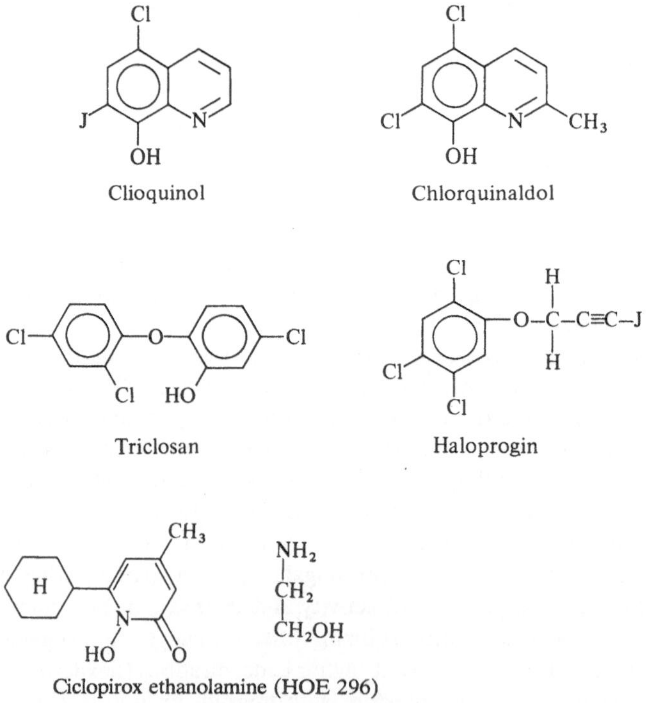

Clioquinol   Chlorquinaldol

Triclosan   Haloprogin

Ciclopirox ethanolamine (HOE 296)

Fig. 41. *Structural formulas of some important broad-spectrum antimicrobials*

Table 18. Minimum inhibitory concentrations (in µg/ml) of haloprogin, clioquinol, chlorquinaldol, triclosan and econazole nitrate for some important types of microorganisms (after [264, 272, 285, 309])

Type of organism	Halo-progin	Clio-quinol	Chlor-quinaldol	Tri-closan	Econazole nitrate
Dermatophytes	1	40	15	10	0.01
Yeasts *(Candida)*	2	10	10	10	12
Molds	15	10	20	100	13
Gram-positive bacteria	2	6	3	0.01	0.01
Gram-negative bacteria	–	40	500	–	–

(– = ineffective)
Salicylic acid would have values of 750, 2000, 2000, 2500, and 3000 for the types of organisms shown. These inhibitory values are far higher than those of the broad-spectrum antimicrobials listed.

The latest development in the area of topically applied antifungals are the imidazole derivatives clotrimazole, miconazole nitrate and econazole nitrate (see Sect. 12). These substances are also active against gram-positive bacteria ("broad-spectrum antimicrobials").

10.7.3 Treatment of Mucous Membrane Mycoses

Only antimycotics with excellent tolerance properties are suitable for use on the mucous membranes. In contrast to the outer skin, the mucous membranes are susceptible mainly to opportunistic mycoses (see Sect. 10.4). Mixed infections with bacteria are often present. For this reason broad-spectrum antimicrobials, and thus substances which are active against bacteria as well as yeasts and molds, are the most effective therapeutic agents.

Special circumstances exist in *vaginitis*. Here the normal saprophytic flora consist of yeasts as well as certain bacteria and protozoa, which may cause disease if overgrowth occurs. Drugs with a narrow spectrum can disturb the microbe balance while exerting no therapeutic effect (overgrowth of other organisms, with little or no change in clinical symptoms).

If we compare the microflora of the healthy and diseased vaginal mucosa, we find that *Candida albicans* occurs 10 times more frequently during disease, trichomonads 18 times more frequently, and bacterioids 20 times more frequently. It should be emphasized once again that the healthy vagina always contains bacterioids, almost always contains *Hemophilus vaginalis (Corynebacterium vaginale)*, often harbors yeasts and rarely contains trichomonads. *Hemophilus vaginalis* is found in 10%–20% of all vaginitis patients (reports range from 6% to 93%), but this organism can be demonstrated in healthy women as well [34]. It is important that the lactobacilli be harmed as little as possible during antimicrobial therapy. Econazole nitrate causes no disturbance of lactobacteria during clinical use [180].

As the lactobacteria increase, the pH falls, normal defense mechanisms are restored, and further antimicrobial actions by chemotherapeutic agents are unnecessary. It should be noted that as the pH falls, the antimicrobial activity of econazole decreases (see Sect. 3.3). Thus, once econazole has exerted its effects, its action will subside by itself. This precludes "overtreatment" phenomena with a disturbance of the microbe balance.

Candidal vaginitis should be treated primarily with drugs which can also prevent the overgrowth of gram-positive bacteria (staphylococci, streptococci), bacterioids, and trichomonads. The imidazole derivative clotrimazole has been tested for its activity against *Hemophilus vaginalis;* a minimum inhibitory concentration of 64 µg/ml was found [92]. Similar activities can be assumed for miconazole and econazole. All imidazole derivatives are active against staphylococci, streptococci, and trichomonads. They thus have a spectrum which guarantees a rapid cure of candidosis, while offering great assurance that no bacterial or trichomonal infection will supervene.

The suspicion that imidazole derivatives with their antibacterial action might damage the physiologic germs in the vagina was dispelled by the results of an experimental investigation: clotrimazole (100 mg in a vaginal tablet) in a treatment course of 6 days produced a marked drop in vaginal physiologic and non physiologic bacteria; on the seventh day after the treatment, however, the normal bacteria generally were as numerous as before [117 a].

11 Systemic Administration of Antimycotically Active Imidazole Derivatives in Man

Clotrimazole, miconazole and econazole can be administered orally or parenterally for the treatment of systemic mycoses in man. The free bases of miconazole and econazole are used in systemic therapy, as opposed to the nitrates used in local therapy.

Clotrimazole leads rapidly to enzyme induction in man and so is no longer used systemically today. Clotrimazole tablets are poorly tolerated, leading to nausea, vomiting, gastric pain, and intestinal complaints (30% of cases). An increase in plasma transaminase activities is observed in 20% of the patients. It has been observed that clotrimazole exerts central nervous effects (5% of cases), and hallucinations may occur. The ability to drive an automobile is impaired [312].

Miconazole is administered orally or intravenously. Miconazole tablets have an unpleasant taste. When administered intravenously, miconazole readily leads to phlebitis, a danger that can be reduced by administering the drug through deeply inserted catheters [296]. Previous therapeutic experience is based on intravenous administrations in doses of about 100–1200 mg [348] three times daily. It is well tolerated, although a reversible, progressive thrombocytosis and anemia are likely to develop with prolonged use [173]. A cardiotoxic reaction was reported in one case [131], in another the occurrence of eruptive xanthomas [25]. The systemic administration of miconazole has proved its worth in the treatment of candidoses of various organs, in mucocutaneous candidoses [40, 167, 327], in systemic mycoses of leukemia patients [303, 309] and after kidney transplantations [342], in pulmonary aspergillosis [117], and in meningitis caused by *Coccidioides immitis* or *Cryptococcus neoformans* [65]. Miconazole can also be administered intrathecally in the treatment of meningitis.

Econazole is supplied in the form of gastric acid-resistant capsules (250 mg). Ampules with 10 mg of the drug for intravenous administration are no longer available. Oral doses of up to 1 g per day are well tolerated by adults. Twice this dose leads to gastrointestinal complaints and central nervous disorders such as dizziness, headache, and auditory and visual disturbances; these changes are rapidly reversible. Econazole is also well tolerated by children when administered in four doses totaling 100 mg/kg daily. When given intravenously, econazole is well tolerated in daily doses up to 600 mg. The systemic administration of econazole has proved suitable for the treatment of chronic mucocutaneous candidosis in children, as well as for the treatment of aspergillosis. It is also effective in the management of urologic infections with *Trichosporon cutaneum* [76]. Experience with maduromycosis has been less encouraging, for the plasma and tissue levels which can be achieved clinically are far below the minimum inhibitory concentrations for *Leptospheria tompkinsii* (32 µg/ml) [76]. In summary, the results obtained with miconazole and econazole have broadened the indications for the systemic treatment of diseases caused by yeasts and molds. In chronic, therapy-resistant dermatomycoses, the systemic administration of miconazole or econazole has been considered in some circumstances in order to prevent the infection from becoming generalized [115]; today, however, ketoconazole is the drug of choice in such cases.

Forms of therapy in which miconazole or econazole are administered alternately with amphotericin B or 5-fluorocytosine have proved quite successful in many cases [336]. Amphotericin B and imidazole derivatives should not be administered concurrently (see Sect. 4.4.6).

Another imidazole derivative R 34 000 (Fig. 6) was only in the testing stage. The oral administration of 1 g in humans leads to serum concentrations which inhibit the growth of *Coccidioides immitis* [162]. R 34 000 will not be developed further. – It seems reasonable to assume that ketoconazole (see Section 2.5.6) will solve the chemotherapeutic problems in systemic mycoses.

To reach a decision as to what kind of a drug should be administered to a patient with a systemic fungal infection, the following considerations apply [54 a]:

If yeasts are isolated, the 5-fluorouracil sensitivity test must be performed; sensitive organisms can be treated with 5-fluorouracil, possibly combined or given alternately with amphotericin B; against partially resistant organisms, amphotericin B must be used together with 5-fluorouracil. In case of a complete resistance, the situation is the same as in cases where no fungal isolate is available: when renal function is normal, amphotericin B may be used depending upon the degree of infection. Due to its side effects, amphotericin B should be administered only to patients with serious infections. In moderate or mild infections, as well as in patients with impaired renal function, the imidazole antifungal ketoconazole is the drug of choice.

Today, with the new compound ketoconazole (cf. Sect. 2. 5. 6) available, the therapeutic situation has improved. This effective and apparently nonnoxious antifungal drug can be administered by the oral route to all patients with systemic infections due to yeasts, yeastlike organisms, and molds. It should be mentioned that ketoconazole may also be used in infections due to dermatophytes; ketoconazole is as effective as griseofulvin in dermatophytosis.

The fact that the treatment of systemic opportunistic mycoses is generally not very promising is due more to the damage already suffered by the host than to a deficiency on the part of the antimycotics administered.

12 Local Application of Antimycotically Active Imidazole Derivatives in Man

12.1 Application to the Outer Skin

The first, relatively low-potency imidazole derivative for the local treatment of dermatomycoses was *chlormidazole* (see Sect. 2.5.2). This substance was used at 2.5% to 5% concentration in ointments, creams and solutions. Chlormidazole was not used on the mucous membranes.

Clotrimazole is applied in the form of a 1% cream for the treatment of dermatomycoses. The high efficacy of this imidazole derivative in dermatomycoses was proved in large-scale double-blind studies. The cure rates for dermatophytoses ranged from 80% (mycoses of the feet) to 98% (mycoses of the body). A cure rate of 92% was reported for candidoses. The cream and solution were about equally effective. Adverse effects (stinging, burning, irritations) were observed in about 3% of the patients treated, probably due to anaphylactoid effects [112, 240, 292, 305, 341]. In tinea cruris, clotrimazole is significantly more effective than haloprogin [319].

Miconazole nitrate is used dermatologically in the form of a cream, powder, solution, and tincture, each with a drug content of 2%. The cure rates correspond to the cure rates for clotrimazole although miconazole possesses superior fungicidal activity. Cures obtained with miconazole are stable. Its tolerance is good [13, 100, 155, 224, 314]; three cases of sensitization have been reported [344]. Even onychomycoses respond to treatment with miconazole of sufficiently long duration [3, 318]. The high efficacy of miconazole in the treatment of skin infections with gram-positive bacteria is emphasized [44, 230].

Econazole nitrate is available for dermatologic use in the form of a cream, solution (spray solution), powder (spray powder) and lotion (skin milk), each with a drug concentration of 1%. Because econazole represents the latest introduction on the market in the area of imidazole derivatives, the results of its clinical use will be discussed in somewhat greater detail.

First let us consider the overall results for two large study populations: In 594 mycosis patients, a cure was effected in 90% of the cases (confirmed by direct examination and culture) with econazole nitrate [282]. In a second large group of 534 patients, a cure rate of 98% was achieved in 282 cases monitored by *culture,* and 89% in 401 cases monitored by *direct examination* [275]. (It should be recalled that dead hyphae can give a false positive result on direct examination.) The above cure rates could be confirmed in smaller groups (50–150 patients) [5, 57, 75, 82, 93, 94, 96, 106, 119, 120, 121, 133, 135, 138, 142, 147, 157, 171, 178, 186, 203, 206, 226, 227, 228, 274, 293, 307, 320, 321, 328]. Good results, even in the case of long-standing mycoses, were emphasized [83]. As expected, checks of clinicochemical indices showed no changes during external econazole therapy [142].

Preparations containing econazole nitrate have also proved effective in the treatment of diseases due to *Pityrosporon* species. Nine cases of follicultitis caused by *Pityrosporon ovale* were quickly and completely cured [72]. With an average treatment time of 3–4 weeks, a cure was effected in 222 of 244 documented cases of pityriasis versicolor [5, 77, 96, 101, 120, 135, 206, 283]. Trichonocardiosis palmellina responds well to topical econazole [154].

French authors used econazole nitrate for the local treatment of 63 patients with severe seborrhea of the face and scalp and an excessive growth of *Pityrosporon ovale*. The cure rate, judged from the clinical picture and the results of microbiologic assays, was 90% [11, 12]. Econazole nitrate also proved effective against tropical mycoses of the skin. The complete cure of epidermophytoses and tokelau was recorded after eight days of treatment [71, 188].

Like miconazole nitrate, econazole nitrate has demonstrated antibacterial activity on topical application. Erythrasma responds well to econazole. For example, 23 of 25 cases were cured with econazole nitrate [12, 75, 135] – an excellent result in view of the chronicity of this disease. For deep skin mycoses, a combination of econazole with retinoic acid was suggested [137].

The rate of adverse effects (burning, etc.) was less than 1% (see Sect. 6.5 and 8.3). In one double-blind study, econazole proved significantly more effective in the treatment of dermatomycoses than clotrimazole [92 a]. When compared to haloprogin, the imidazoles proved to be more active and less irritating [346].

Thus, according to these clinical results, econazole nitrate is to be considered a reliably effective and well-tolerated antimycotic for the treatment of dermatomycoses.

12.2 Application to the Mucous Membranes

In *stomatology*, the imidazole derivatives have proved valuable for the treatment of mycoses in adults as well as children and newborns. For example, miconazole is used in stomatology in the form of lozenges containing 250 mg of the drug. In candidal stomatitis of the denture wearer, the dental prostheses must be soaked for 1 h in a miconazole solution (150 ml with 250 mg miconazole), combined with local treatment of the mucous membranes. Miconazole is up to 100% successful in such applications, although recurrences are frequent [46]. On lesions of the oral cavity, miconazole is used as a 2% oral gel which adheres to the mucous membranes. This presentations form is most useful in babies and children.

In *ophthalmology,* the imidazole derivatives are excellent for the treatment of fungal infections owing to their broad antimicrobial spectrum covering all strains of *Candida, Aspergillus,* and *Fusarium,* and to their good tolerance [141]. Treatment must adhere to an exact schedule, however: applications in 6 h intervals for several weeks are necessary [218].

In *otorhinolaryngology,* a marked increase in fungal infections has been noted, especially in the form of sinusitis and otitis. Of 173 cases of otitis externa, 20% proved to be pure fungal infections, and 5% mixed infections with fungi and bacteria [103]. The fungi most often demonstrated in otitis are *Aspergillus niger* [20] and *Candida albicans.* Less commonly seen are *Penicillium* species, *Cephalosporium* species, and *Scopulariopsis* [21, 103, 136]. *Pityrosporum ovale* can be demonstrated in the human ear in 70%–90% of cases [252]. If the microbial balance is disturbed or inflammatory changes are present, this saprophyte can assume a parasitic role and cause an "opportunistic infection". The use of clotrimazole, miconazole nitrate, and especially econazole nitrate has produced excellent results in the treatment of mycotic otitis [16, 22, 23, 84, 103, 136, 138].

Mycoses are of particularly great importance in *gynecology* (see Sect. 10.5 for discussion). Clotrimazole, miconazole nitrate and econazole nitrate are very effective in the treatment of candidal vaginitis when administered in cream or suppository form. It is apparent that their efficacy is due in part to the broad antimicrobial activity of the imidazole derivatives (Table 19).

When the efficacy of miconazole nitrate (2% cream) was compared with that of nystatin tablets in pregnant women with candidal vaginitis, good clinical results were obtained in both cases. However, negative fungus cultures were

Table 19. Minimum inhibitory concentrations of clotrimazole for bacteria, fungi, and trichomonads (after [287])

Type of organism	Minimum inhibitory concentration in μg/ml[a]
Candida albicans and *Torulopsis glabrata*	0.05– 16
Trichomonas vaginalis	4– 32
Bacterioids (anaerobes)	2– 16
Diplococcus neisserii	64–>256
Staph. aureus	1– 16
Streptococcus faecalis	2– 16
Streptococcus pyogenes	0.5–16
Diphtheroidal bacteria	16–125
Coliform rods *(including Escherichia, Klebsiella* and *Proteus* species)	32–>256
Lactobacteria	125–>256

[a] Concentrations in vaginal fluid after use of a vaginal tablet with 100 mg of the drug: 447 μg/ml after 6–8 h, 57 μg/ml after 10–30 h, and 5 μg/ml after 31–60 h.

found in only 56% of the patients treated with nystatin, while the cultures were negative in 78% of the women given miconazole. Follow-up observations over a period of 3 to 4 months showed a significantly lower recurrence rate among the women treated with miconazole [330].

In another comparative study, miconazole proved to be clearly superior to amphotericin B [332]. Comparisons were also made within the group of imidazole derivatives. Clotrimazole and miconazole nitrate proved to be of approximately equal value in the local treatment of vaginal mycosis [153, 290]. In a more recent study, miconazole was significantly superior to clotrimazole [357]. A direct comparison between econazole and miconazole has not yet been made. – For the treatment of vaginal mycoses, miconazole is used as a 1% cream, as a medicated tampon (100 mg), as a 3-day regime (3 × 400 mg) and as a 7-day regime (7 × 200 mg in gelatine capsules).

The use of *econazole nitrate* in the form of a 1% vaginal cream or in the form of suppositories with 50 mg of the drug produces a cure rate between 90% and 100% in candidal vaginitis [24, 106, 192]. The cream and suppositories are about equally effective [189]. The *permanence* of the cure (assessed both clinically and by negative culture findings) in long-standing, therapy-resistant cases is emphasized [6, 192]. In 1275 documented cases of candidal vaginitis, the vaginal cream produced a complete cure in 1157 patients, for a cure rate of 91% [19, 199, 201, 210, 236, 281, 335]. A second treatment cycle increased the cure rate to 95%–100% [24]. Fourteen-day treatment with suppositories (50 mg daily) led to a cure in 1125 of 1237 patients with vaginal mycosis [51, 132, 184, 200, 201], a cure rate of above 90%. A second treatment cycle increased this rate to 98% [200, 201].

The treatment of candidal vaginitis was greatly simplified by the introduction of *three-day therapy*. In this method a suppository with 150 mg econazole is inserted into the vagina once a day for three days. This three-day cycle was sufficient to effect a complete cure in 1267 of 1452 documented candidal vaginitis cases, for a cure rate of 87% [18, 32, 81, 151, 169, 262]. By adding a second three-day cycle, a cure could be achieved in 98 of 103 patients [32]. The three-day therapy of candidal vaginitis is producing cures which are entirely comparable to those achieved by more prolonged courses of treatment [33, 38, 58, 62, 70, 81, 172, 204]. Beyond this, however, the short course of treatment yields significant advantages in terms of patients compliance, for a short-term treatment is much simpler and more pleasant for the patient. Also, the physician has better assurance that a correct therapeutic schedule will be followed – something that is seldom achieved in 14-day therapy (except in controlled clinical studies). The three-day therapy of candidal vaginitis is well suited to practical conditions and is a welcome development for both patient and physician. – For further data see [350, 351].

The symptoms accompanying candidal vaginitis, such as vulvitis in the patient herself and balanitis in her partner, can be treated with econazole nitrate as a 1% spray powder. A rapid cure could be achieved in 72 of 80 such cases [289].

124

13 Combined Use of Imidazole Derivatives and Glucocorticoids for the Local Treatment of Skin Disease

13.1 Preliminary Remarks

At first sight it may appear contradictory or at least questionable to combine imidazole derivatives or antibiotics with glucocorticoids in local therapy. After all, glucocorticoids possess an immunosuppressive and thus infection-promoting action, which would seem to contraindicate their use in infection.

However, this contraindication applies only to cases in which there is no protection against these actions [235]. The imidazole derivatives, with their broad activity spectrum, that includes gram-positive bacteria, provide such protection in microbial dermatoses.

If clotrimazole, miconazole, or econazole are used together with glucocorticoids, they offer good protection against one of the most frequent adverse effects of the glucocorticoids – the spreading of the infection. They allow glucocorticoids to be used safely (in terms of microbial processes) and successfully on secondarily infected lesions, especially subacute and chronic eczemas.

The use of glucocorticoids is also advantageous in antimicrobial (antifungal) therapy. Intolerance reactions to drugs, preservatives, and bases are prevented (inhibition of sensitivity and hypersensitivity reactions). As the inflammatory process is checked, the normal microflora quickly returns to the skin surface (protection against parasites, see Sect. 9); any overtreatment phenomena (local and even generalized reactions due to the sudden degradation of microorganisms) are avoided. Also, the antipruritic action of the glucocorticoids helps prevent the scratching which can introduce new microorganisms into the lesions.

On the other hand, it must be realized that glucocorticoids can mask infections (the presence of infectious organisms) by suppressing inflammation. Apparent (clinical) healing is followed by a relapse as soon as therapy is halted. However, if a highly active, reliably effective and well-penetrating antimicrobial such as econazole is used in conjunction with the glucocorticoid, the danger of masking is eliminated. It has been shown experimentally that glucocorticoids do not protect the microorganisms from the actions of certain antimicrobials (see below), at least not in the concentration ratio in which the two components are combined.

In contrast to earlier opinions, it is now generally believed that acute "classical" dermatomycoses (dermatophytoses) can be treated with an imidazole derivative combined with a glucocorticoid. The presence of the steroid quickly relieves burning and itching, and subjective symptoms as well as the signs of inflammation disappear more quickly. However, the duration of treatment until the *mycosis is cured* is *not* shortened. This raises the problem of motivating the patient to correctly maintain the treatment for the period of time necessary for complete skin renewal (about 4 weeks). Initial improvement is so rapid that the patient may be tempted to discontinue treatment prematurely. When an antimycotic is prescribed together with a glucocorticoid, the doctor must inform the patient of the necessary duration of treatment in very emphatic terms.

Combined preparations which contain an antimycotic and a glucocorticoid have a permanent place in the external treatment of mycoses [170]. The antimycotic may be an antibiotic or an antimycotically active chemotherapeutic agent with a narrow spectrum or broad spectrum (broad-spectrum antimycotic), or, preferably, a broad-spectrum antimicrobial.

In *acute* lesions, the advantage of glucocorticoids lies in the rapid relief of inflammatory symptoms. In *chronic* mycoses, glucocorticoids prevent lichenification [212] and thus allow the antimycotic to better exert its action.

13.2 Combination of Antibiotics with Glucocorticoids

As prescription figures indicate, preparations combining antibiotics and glucocorticoids have become widely used in local therapy, despite all opposition [166]. Some combinations contain an antibacterially active antibiotic (e. g., neomycin or gentamicin) together with a glucocorticoid; others contain an antifungal antibiotic as well (e. g., natamycin, amphotericin B or nystatin). Combinations of an antifungal antibiotic with a glucocorticoid are rare [1, 2, 166, 233, 254, 326].

It is not easy to demonstrate that such combinations are more effective in the treatment of eczema than the glucocorticoid alone, which can produce good results when applied by itself to certain secondarily infected (colonized) eczemas. Exact judgments are possible only if microbe counts are made. If more than 10^6 staphylococci are present per cm² lesion surface, it will take only a few days for the combination to show its superiority to the monoproduct on the basis of clinical and microbiological evidence [166]. If the counts are low and few staphylococci are present, the combination is no more effective than the pure glucocorticoid preparation. To make the distinction clear, skin areas with few microorganisms are said to be "secondarily infected," or "colonized." If more than 10^6 staphylococci/cm² are present, it is then correct to say that the lesion is "infected." *Clinically,* such a distinction cannot be made. To be on the safe side, therefore, combinations are usually advised. The great need for the local antimicrobial treatment of infected, inflamed skin lesions has been repeatedly and forcefully documented [166].

On secondarily infected *eczemas,* the antibiotic in the combination exerts its full effect only if the microbe count is high [166]. In true *infections,* the gluco-

oid in the combination quickly relieves the subjective symptoms and
ɔtes more rapid healing with no changes in microbiological efficacy. The
iority of a nystatin-triamcinolone combination to nystatin alone has been
nstrated in *Candida* infections [35].

has been shown in pharmacologic tests on humans that the presence of a
ɔorticoid does not hamper the antimicrobial activity of neomycin or nysta-
infections. On the other hand, it has been documented that the presence
ᵹ steroid leads to a rise in the staphylococcal count compared with skin
treated only with ointment base (Table 16).

ᵹfore antibiotics and glucocorticoids are applied together in one prepara-
interactions between them must be ruled out *in vitro*.

ɪe following interactions could conceivably occur:

rect chemical reactions

omotion of degradation or destruction

ɪysicochemical antagonism (common receptor sites)

ɔlogical antagonism (glucocorticoids in low concentrations, such as occur
 deeper skin layers, stimulate the metabolism of *Candida albicans* and
 ɪphylococci; *Pseudomonas aeruginosa* is stimulated at high concentrations
 well, but this is due to the ester radical split off from the glucocorticoid,
 ther than due the glucocorticoid itself, Fig. 24 [231, 232, 233].

fects on penetration (see [69], for example); the *absorption* of the anti-
ɔtic could be inhibited due to the known vascular action of steroids (see
ct. 4.4.4). This effect would be particularly marked at the start of treat-
ᵹnt, since the action of the glucocorticoid decreases after several applica-
ns (tachyphylaxis).

most combinations, interactions between glucocorticoids and antibiotics
 usual concentrations have been ruled out (exceptions: the steroid anti-
 fusidic acid and the highly sterol-reactive heptaene antibiotic hamycin).
 effects of the glucocorticoid on the antimicrobial activity of the antibiotic
 ιled out, it remains to be determined whether the activity of the glucocor-
 is altered by the presence of the antibiotic. The best way to test this is by
 ng the blanching reaction on human skin. So far this test has shown no
 ₅ of antibiotics on the activity of glucocorticoids (more details in [231,
 ₂33, 235, 251]).

₅ antibiotics became less useful in local therapy due to increasing sensiti-
 ι and resistance, therapists focused their interest on the combined use of
 iologically synthesized) chemotherapeutic agents and glucocorticoids.

Salicylic Acid, Haloprogin, Clioquinol, Chlorquinaldol, Friclosan

ombined use of salicylic acid and glucocorticoids lacks antimicrobial ac-
 in the true sense, for the inhibitory concentrations of salicylic acid for

127

microbes (750 µg/ml for *Trichophyton mentagrophytes*, 2000 µg/ml for *Candida albicans* and 2500 µg/ml for staphylococci and streptococci) are too low (see Table 18) to exert adequate effects in deeper skin layers [272]. The clinical tolerance of the drug combination is good. When applied to dry, scaling dermatoses [122], the antimicrobial action of salicylic acid is not utilized so much as its desquamative action. The danger of systemic toxic effects on prolonged administration should be noted.

Haloprogin, chemical name 3-iodo-2-propynyl-2,4,5-trichlorophenyl ether, is combined as needed with a glucocorticoid in the external treatment of microbial dermatoses. The antimicrobial spectrum (activity against gram-negative organisms) of the combination can be broadened by the addition of neomycin. Haloprogin is not influenced antagonistically by neomycin and/or glucocorticoids *in vitro* [246]. The cure rates of haloprogin in the treatment of dermatomycoses are only about 80%, and thus below the cure rates of the imidazole derivatives (cf. lit. [246]). Haloprogin is less effective *in vivo* than *in vitro,* due to the differences in oxygen tension [214].

Clioquinol is used together with flumethasone for the external treatment of microbial and "colonized" dermatoses. There are many favorable reports on the cure rates of such a combination [95, 123, 152].

Chlorquinaldol is also combined with a glucocorticoid for the treatment of dermatoses [39] and dermatomycoses which were superinfected with bacteria. The combination of *triclosan* and flumethasone proved to be equivalent to the combination chlormidazole/fluocinolone acetonide in the treatment of mycoses [261]. Combined applications of the broad-spectrum antimicrobials (haloprogin, clioquinol, chlorquinaldol, triclosan) and glucocorticoids in the local treatment of skin lesions gave good results; no adverse effects attributable to the *combination* were observed (see Sect. 2 and Sect. 10.7.2).

In Table 18 the minimum inhibitory concentrations (mean values for various types of microorganism) of haloprogin, clioquinol, chlorquinaldol, triclosan, and econazole nitrate for dermatophytes, yeasts and bacteria are compared.

13.4 Imidazole Derivatives and Glucocorticoids

So far the imidazoles chlormidazole, clotrimazole, miconazole nitrate, isoconazole nitrate, and econazole nitrate have been used in combination with glucocorticoids for the local treatment of microbial skin lesions.

There are two combinations of chlormidazole: 2.5% chlormidazole with 1% hydrocortisone (as well as 0.05% tyrothricin and 0.3% xanthocillin) and 5% chlormidazole with 0.1% fluocinolone acetonide. The results for dermatomycoses have been entirely favorable, although the steroid does not prevent irritations. The antifungal activity of chlormidazole is somewhat hampered by fluocinolone acetonide *in vitro* [249], but this effect is apparently of no clinical relevance. – Clotrimazole (1%) is applied together with dexamethasone (0.04%) and azidoamphenicol (1%) [347, 358].

Miconazole nitrate is used in dermatological therapy in a concentration of 2% together with 1% hydrocortisone [13, 185, 212] or with 0.25% deperso-lone [310a, 310b]. In double-blind studies the combinations proved superior to the individual components. One study was done over a 4-week period on 63 patients with various fungal or bacterial skin lesions. In the beginning the combination was significantly superior to the 1% hydrocortisone and the 2% miconazole nitrate preparations in its ability to suppress inflammation (rapid amelioration of subjective symptoms). At the conclusion of the test period, 2% miconazole nitrate surpassed the hydrocortisone cream (suppression of inflammation). At the start of treatment, 62 positive microbe cultures were found. In the "combined treatment" group (15 positive for dermatophytes, 6 for bacteria initially), not a single positive dermatophyte or bacterial culture was found after three weeks of treatment. In the miconazole group, the number of positive cultures decreased from 20 to 2; only in the hydrocortisone group (13 positive for dermatophytes, 8 for bacteria initially) were 17 positive cultures still found after three weeks' treatment (11 dermatophyte, 6 bacteria) [185]. Similar good results were reported by another group of authors [91] and could be statistically confirmed [310b].

Isoconazole nitrate (1%) and diflucortolone-21-valerate (0.1%) were combined in a cream and used for the treatment of skin mycoses. In markedly inflammatory and eczematized lesions, the combined preparation was found to be superior in its therapeutic efficacy to the cream containing isoconazole nitrate alone; this observation resulted from a double-blind assay [332a].

Recently, 1% econazole nitrate has been combined with triamcinolone acetonide (0.1%) for the external treatment of dermatoses. One advantage cited in particular is the rapid relief of subjective symptoms associated with microbial lesions. When the corresponding symptoms were evaluated, a statistically significant superiority was found over the preparation without the glucocorticoid [104, 130, 276, 283, 345].

Specifically, it was found that the presence of triamcinolone acetonide did not hamper the therapeutic efficacy of econazole nitrate in the treatment of various forms of tinea. Follow-up culture studies showed the same success rates as the use of econazole nitrate alone. Clinically, however, a more rapid cure was observed. The combined preparation was rated superior to the pure econazole cream by both the attending physician and the patient.

13.5 Indications for the Combined Use of Imidazole Derivatives and Glucocorticoids

Combined preparations can be used in all cases where imidazole derivatives are indicated, and thus on skin infections and secondarily infected (colonized) lesions, whenever marked signs of inflammation are also present.

Clotrimazole, miconazole nitrate, and econazole nitrate are broad-spectrum antimicrobials. They are just as effective, therefore, in the treatment of double infections, atypical infections, and multiple infections as they are in mixed infections. They are particularly valuable in preventing the spread of infections – one of the main adverse effects of glucocorticoids.

The combined use of an imidazole derivative and a glucocorticoid has proved valuable in the treatment of highly inflammatory mycoses, whether caused by dermatophytes, yeasts, or molds (see Sect. 13.4). The use of such combinations has also proved favorable in numerous lesions invaded secondarily by fungi or gram-positive bacteria. Such skin changes occur in many forms: chronic and subacute eczemas (atopic eczema, contact eczema, nummular eczema, etc.), diaper rash, intertriginous eczema, interdigital "mycoses," intertrigo, paronychia, perlèche, cheilitis, balanitis, vulvitis, and otitis. It appears unnecessary to broaden the antimicrobial spectrum of imidazole derivative/ glucocorticoid combinations. The addition of 1% azidoamphenicol to a preparation with 1% clotrimazole and 0.04% dexamethasone increases its activity against gram-positive bacteria, but there is actually no need for this, as controlled studies have shown (see p. 29). Activity against gram-negative organisms is scarcely necessary in the case of eczematous lesions, for these organisms are of no importance in the pathogenesis of inflammatory skin-surface changes (see p. 88).

14 Assessment of Mycoses in Various Branches of Medicine

14.1 Dermatology

Up to 15% of persons seeking dermatologic care suffer from superficial and deep fungal infections, including infections of the nails. According to various statistics, the percentage of dermatologic patients with mycoses varies between 7% and 15%. The dermatophytoses are the classic parasitic mycoses. They are transmitted to man from other persons or from animals. The clinical pictures are typical. Candidoses and diseases caused by molds often present uncharacteristic clinical pictures. These mycoses are regarded as opportunistic infections (see Sect. 9 and 10).

Pityriasis versicolor is the classic saprophytic mysosis. Numerous "tropical" mycoses also affect the skin (cryptococcosis, North American blastomycosis, South American blastomycosis = paracoccidioidomycosis, coccidioidomycosis, histoplasmosis, sporotrichosis, chromomycosis, etc.). For extensive details and photographic documentation, see [61, 126].

14.2 Gynecology

Vaginitis and vulvitis caused by fungi are among the most common diseases in the field of gynecology. These opportunistic fungal infections (see Sect. 10.5) often take an asymptomatic course. In pregnant women, this poses a threat to the newborn infant. Only if signs of the disease are present can treatment be promptly administered to prevent infection of the newborn. For this reason routine checkups and even prophylactic treatment are recommended during pregnancy. The sexual partners of patients with candidal vaginitis and vulvitis contract candidal balanitis in about 50% of the cases.

14.3 Pediatrics

In pediatrics, both dermatomycoses and the sometimes serious consequences of neonatal infections must be dealt with. The latter may be manifested simply as candidal stomatitis, or may lead to a chronic enteritis. Many obstinate diaper rash cases are due to candidoses. Only after the intestinal tract is degermed can treatment of the skin bring a lasting cure. Systemic "opportunistic" mycoses are indicative of immunologic defects.

14.4 Stomatology

Candidal stomatitis is the most frequent disease accompanying the wearing of dentures. General factors are of less importance in the occurrence of "opportunistic" fungal infection than are local factors such as improper hygiene or poorly fitting dentures (see Sect. 10.4.1). In life-threatening diseases of the immune system (leukemias) and carcinomas, every fifth patient contracts oral candidosis (candidal stomatitis) during the final 8 weeks of life.

14.5 Otorhinolaryngology

Inflammatory diseases of the middle ear and external auditory canal often exhibit invasion by fungi. A search for the presence of fungi is now routine in external auditory canal changes [85]. Opportunistic fungal infections must also be suspected in chronic paranasal sinusitis.

14.6 Ophthalmology

An increase in fungal infections has also been observed in ophthalmology. Often the opportunistic mycosis caused by *Candida, Fusarium,* or *Aspergillus* species can be traced to the improper use of glucocorticoid-containing preparations or to long-term antibiotic therapy. Keratomycoses lead to permanent visual disturbances and can even cause blindness.

14.7 Proctology

The importance of the fungi (mainly yeasts from the bowel) in pruritus ani and anal eczemas is often underrated. Chronic anal eczemas are extremely prone to opportunistic invasion (and clinical exacerbation) by fungi [260]. In every third person, yeasts and/or molds inhabit the anorectal region as saphrophytes [187].

In patients with anorectal complaints, *Candida albicans* is present in the rectum in about 40% of the cases.

14.8 Urology

The increase in candidal vaginitis and candidal balanitis has been paralleled by a marked increase in the incidence of candidal urethritis and candidal cystitis. Urethritis which is treated excessively with various antibiotics is frequently superseded by candidal urethritis. In this case antibiotic therapy is of prime pathogenic importance for the "opportunistic" mycosis. It is known, for example, that patients with "psychic" urethritis (guilt feelings, lesion of the urethra by constant expression) go from doctor to doctor to receive a continual supply of new antibiotics.

Fungi can be introduced into the urogenital tract through catheters, which may cause severe infection in patients whose defenses are impaired. Kidney transplantations may be followed by opportunistic fungal infections due to the cytostatics which are given postoperatively. These suppress the immune response not only to the foreign tissue, but also to fungi.

14.9 Internal Medicine

Practically all the internal organs are susceptible to opportunistic fungal infection. Candidal endocarditis presents particular diagnostic problems.

Mycotic diseases of the gastrointestinal tract (esophagitis, enteritis) occur on depression of the immune response or under heavy antibiotic therapy. These are mycoses of internal surfaces. Safe and effective therapeutic agents are available.

Besides direct mycotic infections, diseases resulting from hypersensitivity to certain fungi must also be dealt with in internal medicine [4]. The role of fungi as respiratory allergens in the genesis of bronchial asthma and vasomotor rhinitis is also noted.

14.10 Orthopedics

Mycotic arthritis can occur as a symptom of systemic candidoses. Invasion of the bone has also been observed in aspergillosis.

14.11 Surgery, Intensive Care, Anesthesiology

Patients in need of intensive care are extremely susceptible to opportunistic fungal infections. There is a good chance that such infections will be introduced by catheters and various other devices, and sometimes they are practically unavoidable.

15 Concluding Remarks

The imidazole derivatives have substantially broadened and enhanced possibilities for the local antimycotic treatment of the skin and mucous membranes. A final judgment cannot yet be made on the systemic administration of the imidazole derivatives. Further studies and observations are necessary, and perhaps imidazole derivatives other than those now available will one day solve the problems still associated with the treatment of systemic mycoses due to yeasts and molds. Today, the situation looks most promising with ketoconazole, an imidazole derivative active upon oral administration.

When administered locally, the imidazole derivatives do offer many advantages. Their antimicrobial spectrum covers all fungi pathogenic to man, as well as gram-positive bacteria; they also protect against an overgrowth of trichomonads. The clinical pharmacologic properties of the imidazole derivatives permit their risk-free use. They are almost entirely devoid of adverse effects (practically no sensitization, no photoallergic or phototoxic effects, very low anaphylactoid activity). Their good penetration and high antimicrobial activity make it possible to combat infection in deeper skin layers; even in the dermis, microbistatic concentrations are achieved. The penetration of econazole nitrate is particularly good. This fact, plus its very high antimicrobial activity, is why econazole nitrate is considered in all fields of medicine to be an excellent drug for use on the skin and mucous membranes.

The broad antimicrobial spectrum of the imidazole derivatives clotrimazole, miconazole, isoconazole, and econazole ensures a reliable therapeutic activity even in cases where the clinical picture and direct microscopic evidence do not allow the pathogen to be identified, or when several types of microorganism are present. Moreover, the antibacterial activity of these drugs prevents the overgrowth of individual strains due to a disturbance of the microbe balance or proliferation *in vacuo*.

In gynecology, the activity of the imidazole derivatives against fungi, bacteria and trichomonads has proved to be highly beneficial in the treatment of vaginal mycosis. In this case the use of chemotherapeutic agents with a narrow spectrum readily leads to the overgrowth of other strains and thus to therapeutic failure, at least in a clinical sense. With the imidazole derivatives, this danger is avoided.

16 References

1 Abdel Aal, H., Abdel Fattah, A., El Shiemy, S., Faris, R., Tadros, S. S.: A double-blind comparison of a new combination (halcinonide-neomycin-amphotericin) and active controls in cutaneous candidiasis and steroid-responsive dermatoses. J. Int. Med. Res. **4**, 232–236 (1976)

2 Abdel Aal, H., Tadros, S. S.: Treatment of steroid-responsive dermatoses. An assessment of halcinonide-neomycin-nystatin (HNN). Clin. Trials J. **13**, 118–123 (1976)

3 Achten, G., Degreef, H., Dockx, P.: Treatment of onychomycosis with a solution of miconazole 2% in alcohol. Mykosen **20**, 251–256 (1977)

4 Almog, C. H., Beemer, A. M., Kuttin, E. S.: Allergic respiratory disease associated with Candida and Trichophyton. Castellania **5**, 181–183 (1977)

5 Amblard, P.: L'éconazole et le traitement des mycoses en dermatologie. Rev. méd. Alpes franç. **6**, 41–43 (1977)

6 Anger, H.: Neue Therapiemöglichkeiten vulvovaginaler Mykosen: Klinische Studie zur Feststellung der optimalen Therapiedauer mit Econazol-nitrat Vaginalcrème. Symposion über Econazol-nitrat, Boppard/Rhein 1977, pp. 77–78 Melsungen: Notabene Medici 1978

7 Anséhn, S.: In vitro synergistic action of antimycotics and antibiotics on Candida albicans. Curr. Ther. Res. **22**, 92–99 (1977)

8 Anséhn, S., Boqvist, L., Schönebeck, J., Winblad, B.: Effect of antimycotics in the surface morphology of Candida albicans. Castellania **2**, 41–44 (1974)

9 Anséhn, S., Winblad, B.: Surface morphology of Candida albicans after treatment with antimycotic drugs. Int. Symposium Medical Mycology, Flims 1977. Mykosen, Suppl. 1, 322–327 (1978)

10 Arcy, P. F., Scott, E. M.: Antifungal agents. Progr. Drug Res. **1978**, 93–147

11 Aron-Brunetière, R., Dompmartin-Pernot, D., Drouhet, E.: Le traitement du pityriasis capitis (état pelliculaire) par le nitrate d'éconazole. Rev. Méd. (Paris) **17**, 1285–1290 (1976)

12 Aron-Brunetière, R., Dompmartin-Pernot, D., Drouhet, E.: Treatment of pityriasis capitis (dandruff) with econazole nitrate. Acta derm.-venereol. (Stockh.) **57**, 77–80 (1977)

13 Aussems, J.: Clinical evaluation of miconazole tincture in skin mycoses. Mykosen **20**, 269–272 (1977)

14 Aussems, J., Van Cutsem, J.: Traitment des lésions dermatologiques au Dactacort. Ars. Méd. (Bruxelles) **29**, 2187–2193 (1974)

15 Avram, A., Grupper, Ch.: Un nouvel antifongique à large spectre: l'éconazole. Action in vitro et in vivo. Bull. Soc. Franç. Mycol. Méd. **4**, 2 (1975)

16 Avram, A., Grupper, Ch.: Essais concernant l'activité antifongique et antibacterienne "in vitro" de l'éconazole. 6th Congress ISHAM, Tokyo, 1975

17 Ayliffe, G. A. J., Green, W., Livingston, R., Lowbury, E. J. L.: Antibiotic-resistant Staphylococcus aureus in dermatology and burn wards. J. clin. Path. **30**, 40–44 (1977)

18 Balmer, J. A.: Three-day therapy of vulvovaginal candidiasis with econazole: A multicentric study comprising 996 cases. Amer. J. Obstet. Gynec. **126**, 436–441 (1976)

19 Balmer, J. A.: Vaginale Candidiasis und ihre Behandlung mit Econazol. Ars. Med. (Liestal) **66**, 195–197 (1976)

20 Bambule, J., Grigoriu, D.: L'aspergillose sinusale. Bull. Soc. Mycol. Med. **5**, 181–184 (1976)

21 Bambule, J., Grigoriu, D.: Les otomycoses. Bull. Soc. Mycol. Méd. **6**, 71–74 (1977)

22 Bambule, J., Grigoriu, D.: Otomycoses and their treatment. International Symposium Medical Mycology, Flims 1977. Mykosen, Suppl. 1, 82–86 (1978)

23 Bambule, J., Grigoriu, D.: Fungal nasosinusitis treated with econazole. International Symposium Medical Mycology, Flims 1977. Mykosen, Suppl. 1, 87–93 (1978)

24 Bardiaux, M., Bonhomme, J., Crimail, Ph., Darmon, M., Guillaumin, J.-P., Julien-Laferrière, P., Le Lièvre, H., Le Louet, J.-M., Leroy, B., Martin-Dupray, D., Torre, M.-Ph.: Nouvel apport dans le traitement des mycoses vulvo-vaginales: l'éconazole. Sem. Hôp. (Paris) **52**, 493–499 (1976)

25 Barr, R. J., Fujita, W. H., Graham, J. H.: Eruptive xanthomas associated with intravenous miconazole therapy. Arch. Dermatol. **114**, 1544–1545 (1978)

26 Bartmann, K.: Antimikrobielle Chemotherapie. Berlin-Heidelberg-New York: Springer 1974

27 Bartmann, K., Plempel, M.: Neue Testmethoden in der Mykologie. Münch. med. Wschr. **118**, Suppl. 1, 6–11 (1976)

28 Bauer, R., Raff, W. K.: Stand der heutigen Antimykotika-Therapie. Castellania **5**, 209–213 (1977)

29 Baumgart, G., Stelzl, G.: Auswirkungen von Ultraschallbehandlung auf den imperfekten Pilz Scopulariopsis brevicaulis und seine Pathogenität. Castellania **4**, 41–43 (1976)

30 Bayot, D.: Essai en clinique gynécologique d'un nouveau traitement local de la vaginite. Brux. Méd. **54**, 515–517 (1974)

31 Becker, H.: Experimentelle pharmakologische und toxikologische Untersuchungen mit Econazol-nitrat. Symposion über Econazol-nitrat, Boppard/Rhein 1977, pp. 21–28. Melsungen: Notabene Medici 1978

32 Beeguer, J.: Un traitement de trois jours des candidiases vaginales. Méd. et Hyg. (Genève) **34**, 1925–1927 (1976)

33 Belaisch, J., Cohen, J., Dupay, A., Hervet, E., Hewitt, J., Netter, A., Ravina, J. H., Sureau, C.: Le traitement de 3 jours des mycoses vulvo-vaginales. Une innovation en thérapeutique gynécologique. Gynécologie **28**, 557–561 (1977)

34 Bergman, S., Lundgren, K. M.: Haemophilus vaginalis in vaginitis. Acta obstet. gynec. scand. **44**, 8–17 (1965)

35 Beveridge, G. W., Fairburn, E., Finn, O. A., Scott, O. L. S., Stewart, T. W., Summerly, R.: A comparison of nystatin cream with nystatin/triamcinolone acetonide combination cream in the treatment of candidal inflammation of the flexures. Curr. med. Res. Opin. **4**, 584–587 (1977)

36 Bhargava, A. S., Staben, P., Nieuweboer, B., Guenzel, P.: Effect of hexachlorophene on the coagulation process in beagle dogs. Arzneimittel-Forsch. **26**, 2183–2185 (1976)

37 Bibel, D. J., Lovell, D. J.: Skin flora maps: tool in study of cutaneous ecology. J. invest. Derm. **67**, 265–269 (1976)

38 Bilharino, M. R., Barbosa de Souza, H.: Estudo clinico do econazole na terapeutica das vulvovaginites micoticas. Folha Méd. **74**, 253–256 (1977)

39 Blair, C., Dainow, I. I.: Clinical experiences with a new steroid-antibacterial preparation in the treatment of infected eczema. A pilot study in twenty-eight patients. Brit. J. clin. Pract. **32**, 289–290 (1978)

40 Blomqvist, K., Horsmanheimo, M.: Systemic miconazole treatment of a patient with chronic granulomatous mucocutaneous candidiasis. Acta derm.-venereol. **58**, 455–459 (1978)

41 Borelli, D., Bran, J. L., Fuentes, J., Legendre, R., Leiderman, E., Levine, H. B., Restrepo, A., Stevens, D. A.: Ketoconazole, an oral antifungal: laboratory and clinical assessment of imidazole drugs. Postgrad. Med. J. (in press)

42 Bork, K.: Die Kontaktdermatitis. Med. Welt **27**, 1923–1925 (1976)

43 Bortolussi, R. A., Bannatyne, R. M., Arbus, G. S.: Treatment of Candida peritonitis by peritoneal lavage with amphotericin B. J. Pediat. **87**, 987–988 (1975)

44 Botter, A. A.: Further experiences with miconazole nitrate, a broadspectrum antimycotic with antibacterial activity. Mykosen **15**, 179–183 (1972)

44a Botter, A. A., Dethier, F., Mertens, R. L., Morias, J., Peremans, W.: Skin and nail mycoses: treatment with ketoconazole, a new oral antimycotic agent. Mykosen **22**, 274–278 (1979)

45 Bradford, L. G., Montes, L. F.: Perioral dermatitis and Candida albicans. Arch. Derm. **105**, 892–895 (1972)

46 Brincker, H.: Treatment of oral candidiasis in debilitated patients with miconazole – a new potent antifungal drug. Scand. J. infect. Dis. **8**, 117–120 (1976)

47 Brodie, R. R., Chasseaud, L. F., Walmsley, L. M.: High-performance liquid chromatographic determination of the antimycotic agent econazole in plasma. J. Chromatogr. **155**, 209–213 (1978)

48 Brotherton, J.: Biological assay of fungicides against yeasts in vitro using a coulter counter. Mykosen **19**, 361–372 (1976)

49 Brown, J., Wannamaker, L. W., Ferrieri, P.: Enumeration of β-haemolytic Streptococci on normal skin by direct agar contact. J. med. Microbiol. **8**, 503–512 (1975)

50 Brugmans, J., Van Cutsem, J., Heykants, J., Schuermans, V., Thiepont, D.: Systemic antifungal potential, safety, biotransport and transformation of miconazole nitrate. Europ. J. clin. Pharmacol. **5**, 93–96 (1972)

51 Callies, R.: Erfahrungen bei der Behandlung der Soor-Kolpitis mit Econazol-nitrat. Symposion über Econazol-nitrat, Boppard/Rhein 1977, pp. 71–76. Melsungen: Notabene Medici 1978

52 Cameron, B. D., Chasseaud, L. F., Conway, B., Fox, N., Taylor, T.: Absorption and disposition of econazole nitrate after application to the skins and vaginas of rabbits. Arzneimittel-Forsch. **26**, 2054–2059 (1976)

53 Cartwright, R. Y.: Pharmacology of imidazole derivatives with antimycotic activity. Int. Symposium Medical Mycology, Flims 1977, Mykosen, Suppl. 1, 298–303 (1978)

54 Cartwright, R. Y.: Absorption of econazole from the human gastrointestinal tract. Curr. Chemother. **1978**, 231–233

55 Cartwright, R. Y.: Econazole. In vitro and in vivo studies. VIIth Congress of the International Society for Human and Animal Mycology, Tel Aviv, March 1979

56 Chappel, C.: Absorption, metabolism and excretion of H^3-econazole (base) in the cynomolgus monkey. Bio Research Laboratories, Montreal, Research Report No. 8496/1, 1974

57 Chin, H. S., Kim, J. H.: A clinical study on the treatment of dermatomycosis with econazole nitrate (Pevaryl) cream. New med. J. **21**, 75–80 (1978)

58 Choi, I. B.: Three days therapy of fungal vaginitis with econazole nitrate vaginal suppository 150 mg. New med. J. **21**, 51–54 (1978)

59 Costa, A. L., Valenti, A., Loteta, L. E., Midili, S.: Antimycotic activity of miconazole (R 18134) in vitro and in vito. Mykosen **20**, 431–440 (1977)

60 Dean, A. V., Lan, S. J., Kripalani, K. J., DiFazio, L. T.: Metabolism of ^{14}C-econazole nitrate in monkeys. Fed. Proc. **36**, 938 (1977)

61 Delacrétaz, J., Grigoriu, D., Ducel, G.: Color atlas of medical mycology. Bern-Stuttgart-Vienna: Huber 1976

62 De Luca, L. A., Ridrigues, J. R., Berezowsky, A. T., Torres de Sa, T.: Terapeutica da candidiase vaginal com econazole – novo antimicotico topico de amplo espectro. J. Bras. Gin. **83**, 95–98 (1977)

63 De Nollin, S., Borgers, M.: The ultrastructure of Candida albicans after in vitro treatment with miconazole. Sabouraudia **12**, 341–351 (1974)

64 De Nollin, S., Borgers, M.: An ultrastructural and cytochemical study of Candida albicans after in vitro treatment with imidazoles. Mykosen **19**, 317–328 (1976)

65 Deresinski, S. C., Lilly, R. B., Levine, H. B., Galgiani, J. N., Stevens, D. A.: Treatment of fungal meningitis with miconazole. Amer. Rev. resp. Dis. **113**, 71 (1976)

66 Dittmar, W., Grau, W.: Ciclopirox – Substanz mit Aspekten für Mykologie und Kosmetik. Ärztl. Kosmetologie **9**, 209–214 (1979)

66a Dittmar, W., Lohaus, G.: HOE 296, a new antimycotic compound with a broad antimicrobial spectrum. Arzneimittel-Forsch. **23**, 670–674 (1973)

67 Dixon, D., Shadomy, S., Shadomy, H. J., Expinel-Ingroff, A.: Comparison of the in vitro antifungal activities of miconazole and a new imidazole, R 41 400. J. infect. Dis. **138**, 245–248 (1978)

68 Dobias, B.: Specific and non-specific immunity in Candida infections. Acta med. scand. Suppl. **421**, 1–94 (1964)

69 Dobozy, A., Peter, S., Simon, N.: Die Wirkung von Steroidverbindungen auf die perkutane Resorption einiger Antibiotika. Hautarzt, Suppl. **1**, 11–14 (1976)

70 Dogniez, B., Sandrot-Degee, M. A., Lambotte, R.: Experimentation clinique de l'éconazole en ovules vaginaux à 150 mg dans la candidose vaginale. Acta Therapeutica **4**, 119–124 (1978)

71 Dompmartin, D., Drouhet, E.: Folliculites à Pityrosporum ovale. Action de l'éconazole. Bull. Soc. Mycol. Méd. **6**, 15–20 (1977)

72 Dompmartin, D., Drouhet, E., Moreau, E.: Nouvelle enquéte sur "tinea imbricata" (tokelau) et autres épidermomycoses tropicales en Océanie (Iles Nouvelles-Hebrides et Banks); résultats favorables avec un nouvel antifongique, "éconazole" en traitement local. Bull. Soc. Franç. Derm. Syph. **82**, 422–427 (1975)

73 Dorn, M., Roehnert, K.: Scanning electron microscopy of Pityrosporum furfur. Int. Symposium Medical Mycology, Flims, 1977. Mykosen, Suppl. 1, 141–145 (1978)

74 Dorn, M., Russwurm. R.: Tierexperimentelle Untersuchungen zur Beeinflussung der Wundheilung durch Candida albicans. Arch. Derm. Res. **256**, 205–212 (1976)

75 Dorn, M., Scherwitz, Ch., Lentze, I., Plewig, G.: Econazol-nitrat. In-vitro-Testung und klinische Prüfung. Münch. med. Wschr. **117**, 687–692 (1975)

76 Drouhet, E., Dupont, B.: Preliminary studies on the pharmacology and therapeutic activity of oral and intravenous econazole. Int. Symposium Med. Mycology, Flims 1977. Mykosen, Suppl. 1, 192–201 (1978)

77 Drouhet, E., Dompmartin, D., Papachristou-Moraiti, A.: Pathogenic capacities of Pityrosporum ovale and/or P. orbiculare in experimental animals and humans. VIIth Congress of the International Society for Human and Animal Mycology, Tel Aviv, March 1979

78 Duhm, B., Maul, W., Medenwald, M., Patzschke, K., Wegener, L. A., Oberste-Lehn, M.: Pharmakokinetik nach topischer Anwendung von Bisphenyl-(2-chlorphenyl)-1-imidazolyl-methan-(^{14}C). Arzneimittel-Forsch. **22**, 1276–1280 (1972)

79 Duhm, B., Medenwald, M., Puetter, J., Maul, W., Patzschke, K., Wegener, L. A.: The pharmacokinetics of clotrimazole-^{14}C. Postgrad. med. J. **50**, 13–17 (1975)

80 Dupont, B., Drouhet, E.: Synergy and antagonism of antifungal agents. VIIth Congress of the International Society for Human and Animal Mycology, Tel Aviv, March 1979

81 Ebert, H.: Die Kurztherapie vulvovaginaler Mykosen mit Econazol-nitrat. Symposion über Econazol-nitrat, Boppard/Rhein 1977, pp. 65–69. Melsungen: Notabene Medici 1978

82 Editorial Note: Parenteral treatment with imidazole antimycotics. Curr. med. Res. Opin. **5**, 365 (1978)

83 Eichmann, Th.: Lokale Behandlung von Pilzaffektionen der Haut mit Econazol, einem neuen Breitspektrum-Antimykotikum. Schweiz. Rundsch. Med. (Praxis) **63**, 719–721 (1974)

84 Elbaz, P.: Etude de l'efficacité et de la tolérance du Pevaryl lait 1% dans le traitement des mycoses du conduit auditif externe. Ann. Otolaryngol. **1978**, 315–320

85 El-Gothamy, M. A. B., El-Gothamy, Z.: Otomycosis – a new line of treatment. Castellania **5**, 215–216 (1977)

86 Elkhouly, A. E.: Verfügbarkeit von Nystatin aus verschiedenen Dermatica gegen Candida albicans. Mykosen **19**, 227–237 (1976)

87 Ferry, D. G., Roberts, M. T. S., Otago, N., Dunedin, Z.: Hexachlorophene absorption in premature infants and surgical patients. Clin. exp. Pharmacol. Physiol. **4**, 211 (1977)

88 Feuerman, E., Alteras, I.: The prevalence of mycotic infections and the immunologic response in patients with housewives' eczema. Mykosen **19**, 51–54 (1972)

89 Fischer, T., Hartvig, P.: Skin absorption of 8-hydroxyquinolines. Lancet **1977/I**, 603

90 Fischer, T., Fagerlund, C., Hartvig, P.: Absorption of 8-hydroxyquinolines through the human skin. Acta derm.-venereol. (Stockh.) **58**, 407–411 (1978)

91 Fischman, O., Levites, J., Grinblat, M.: Daktacort in skin lesions. Mykosen **20**, 471–475 (1977)

92 Förster, D., Melchior, K., Plempel, M., Schnell, J. D.: Canesten-Wirkung auf Haemophilus vaginalis (Corynebacterium vaginale). Münch. med. Wschr. **118**, Suppl 1, 53–55 (1976)

92a Fredriksson, T.: Treatment of dermatomycoses with topical econazole and clotrimazole. Curr. ther. Res. **25**, 590–594 (1979)

93 Garrel, J., Millet, P., Jeanney, J. C., Jaquelin, R.: Un nouvel antimycosique d'action polyvalente: l'éconazole. Résultats thérapeutiques. Méd. arm. **4**, 1–5 (1976)

94 Gauthier, O., Texier, M. L.: Un nouveau fongicide polyvalent: L'éconazole dans le traitment des mycoses cutanées. Bordeaux médical **11**, 227–229 (1978)

95 Gip, L.: Betamethasone dipropionate ointment with chinoform and betamethasone valerate ointment with chinoform. A double-blind comparison in secondarily infected dermatoses. Curr. ther. Res. **24**, 630–632 (1978)

96 Gisslen, H., Hersle, K., Mobacken, H., Nordin, P.: Topical treatment of dermatomycoses and tinea versicolor with econazole cream 1% (Pevaryl®). Curr. ther. Res. **21**, 681–684 (1977)

97 Gloor, M., Geilhof, A., Ronneberger, G., Friedrich, H. C.: Biochemical and physiological parameters on the healthy skin surface of persons with candidal intertrigo and of persons with tinea cruris. Arch. Derm. Res. **257**, 203–211 (1976)

98 Götz, H.: Neuere Befunde über Hautkrankheiten durch Dermatophyten. Münch. med. Wschr. **120**, 1379–1382 (1978)

99 Götz, H., Bever, U.: Beobachtungen über Dermatophytenbefall bei der Neurodermitis constitutionalis. Mykosen **20**, 107–111 (1977)

100 Götz, H., Zabel, M.: Unterschwellige Röntgenstrahlendosen als akzidenteller infektionsfördernder Faktor für eine Tinea des rechten Zeigefingers. Mykosen **20**, 224–228 (1977)

101 Grigoriu, D.: Aspects cliniques, histologiques et thérapeutiques du pityriasis versicolor. Bull. Soc. Mycol. Méd. **6**, 25–28 (1977)

102 Grigoriu, D.: Medicaments antifongiques actuels. Mycoses superficielles. Schweiz. Rundschau Med. (Praxis) **66**, 871–874 (1977)

103 Grigoriu, D., Bambule, J., Savary, M., Delacrétaz, J.: Sinusite frontale fongique. VIIthe Congress of the International Society for Human and Animal Mycology, Tel Aviv, March 1979

104 Grigoriu, D., Grigoriu, A.: Etude thérapeutique des mycoses superficielles. Bull. Soc. Mycol. Méd. **6**, 295–299 (1977)

105 Grigoriu, D., Grigoriu, A.: Herpes circiné par Microsporum gypseum et M. cookei. Bull. Soc. Mycol. Méd. **6**, 129–132 (1977)

106 Grigoriu, A., Grigoriu, D.: Herpes circiné provoqué par Tr. rodhaini? (Variante africaine du Tr. rubrum). Bull. Soc. Mycol. Méd. **7**, 89–92 (1978)

107 Grigoriu, A., Grigoriu, D.: Study of the antifungal capacity by means of the contact test. Arzneimittel-Forsch. **29**, 569–571 (1979)

107a Grimmer, H.: Systemic use of the imidazoles in dermatology/gynecology. Round Table Discussion on the therapeutic Use of Oral Econazole. Zurich, June 1979

107b Gründer, K., Petzold, D.: Der Einfluß eines Kortikosteroidzusatzes auf das Ergebnis der Lokalbehandlung der bakteriell superinfizierten Tinea pedum intertriginosa. Hautarzt **30**, 392–395 (1979)

108 Grupper, Ch., Avram, A.: Un nouvel antifongique à large spectre: l'éconazole. Action in vitro et in vivo. 6th Congress ISHAM, Tokyo 1975

109 Guez, C., Tourne, C. E., Ritter, J., Gandar, R.: Etude de l'action du Gyno-Pévaryl® sur les mycoses génitales. Méd. Nord et Est, 1976, **11**, 1–3 (1976)

110 Haller, I.: Vergleichende experimentelle Prüfung moderner Antimykotika in vitro und in vivo. Hautarzt **28**, Suppl. 2, 187–188 (1977)

111 Haller, I., Plempel, M.: Experimental in vitro and in vivo comparison of modern antimycotics. Curr. Med. Res. Opin. **5**, 315–327 (1977/78)

112 Haller, I.: Imidazole antimycotis: Experience with clotrimazole, experimental aspects, aims for the future. Abstracts XII. International Congress Microbiology, Munich, Sept. 1978, Nr. 38/3

113 Haller, I., Mendling, W.: Sind bei der Strahlentherapie von Genitalkarzinomen der Frau Nebenwirkungen auf eine vorhandene vaginale Sprosspilzflora – insbesondere das Auftreten resistenter Mutanten – zu fürchten? Mykosen **21**, 313–317 (1978)

114 Hansson, H.: Mycotic infections in eczematous patients. Curr. ther. Res. **22**, 24–26 (1977)

115 Hantschke, D., Wente, W., Gronemann, A.: Paronychie durch Aspergillus flavus Link. Mykosen **20**, 122–126 (1977)

116 Hantschke, D.: In vitro sensitivity tests with antimycotic imidazole derivatives and evaluation of results. International Symposium Medical Mycology, Flims, 1977. Mykosen, Suppl. 1, 222–229 (1978)

117 Hantschke, D., Schulte, R., Dabag, S., Greschuna, D.: Treatment with econazole of a case of pulmonary aspergillosis. International Symposium Medical Mycology, Flims, 1977. Mykosen, Suppl. 1, 230–235 (1978)

117a Hantschke, D., Zabel, M.: The reaction of the physiological vaginal flora to topical antimycotics. Mykosen **22**, 267–273 (1979)

118 Heel, R. C., Brogden, R. N., Speight, T. M., Avery, G. S.: Econazole: a review of its antifungal activity and therapeutic efficacy. Drugs **16**, 177–201 (1978)

119 Heinke, E.: Erfahrungen mit Econazol-nitrat bei der Behandlung dermaler Mykosen in einer dermatologischen Praxis. Symposion über Econazol-nitrat, Boppard/ Rhein 1977, pp. 125–126. Melsungen: Notabene Medici 1978

120 Hempel, M.: Klinische Erfahrungen in der lokalen Behandlung von Dermatomykosen mit Econazol-Hautmilch. Mykosen **18**, 213–219 (1975)

121 Hempel, M. B.: Klinische Prüfung von Econazol-Spraylösung und -Spraypuder bei Hautmykosen. Z. Hautkr. **53**, 935–939 (1978)

122 Herz, G.: Modernes Kortikoid-Kombinationsexternum für die pädiatrische Dermatotherapie. Ärztl. Prax. **24**, 483–486 (1972)

123 Herz, G.: Kortikoidexterna in der pädiatrischen Praxis. München: Marseille 1973

124 Herz, G.: Therapie und Mikrobiologie infizierter Dermatosen beim Kind. Ärztl. Prax. **26**, 3433–3439 (1974)

125 Herz, G.: Bacterial flora of the healthy skin in children. J. int. Med. Res. **4**, 367–374 (1976)

126 Hildick-Smith, G., Blank, H., Sarkany, I.: Fungus diseases and their treatment. Boston: Little & Brown 1964

127 Holt, R. J.: Topical pharmacology of imidazole antifungals. J. cutan. Pathol. **3**, 45–59 (1976)

128 Holt, R. J., Newman, R. L.: The treatment of urinary candidosis with the oral antifungal drugs 5-fluorocytosine and clotrimazole. Develop. Med. Child Neurol. **14**, Suppl. 27, 70–76 (1973)

129 Holt, R. J., Azmi, A.: Miconazole-resistant Candida. Lancet **1978/I**, 50–51

130 Huber, H. P.: Behandlung entzündlicher Dermatomykosen mit Pevisone und Pevaryl. Schweiz. Rundschau Med. (Praxis) **68**, 92–96 (1979)

131 Huijgens, P. C., Boeijinga, J. K., Van der Meer, J.: Een mogelijk cardiotoxische reactie van miconazole-injectiev-loeistof. Ned. T. Geneesk. **119**, 1549–1551 (1975)

132 Hur, M., Kim, D. H.: The clinical effects of econazole nitrate vaginal suppository for candidal vaginitis. J. Res. Inst. Med. Sci. Korea **9**, 71–75 (1977)

133 Huriez, Cl., Thomas, P.: Le Pevaryl® en dermatologie (à propos de 30 observations). Lille méd. **22**, 272–274 (1977)

134 Ippen, H.: Einfache in-vitro-Untersuchungen zur photodynamischen und photoallergischen Reaktion. Arch. klin. exp. Derm. **237**, 499–501 (1970)

135 Itani, Z. S.: Über die Zunahme der Mykosen in Deutschland. Erfahrungen mit dem neuen Breitband-Antimykotikum Econazol. Z. Haut. u. Geschl.-Kr. **49**, 683 (1974)

136 Itani, Z. S.: Die Behandlung der Otomykosen mit dem neuen Breitband-Antimykotikum Econazol. Mykosen **19**, 247–250 (1976)

137 Itani, Z. S.: Dermatophytes contracted from animals. International Symposium Medical Mycology, Flims, 1977. Mykosen, Suppl. 1, 108–111 (1978)

138 Itani, Z. S.: Über die Zunahme der Mykosen in Deutschland. Erfahrungen mit dem neuen Breitband-Antimykotikum Econazol-nitrat bei der Behandlung von Dermatomykosen und Otomykosen. Symposium über Econazol-Nitrat, Boppard/ Rhein, pp. 101–111. Melsungen: Notabene Medici 1978

139 Iwata, K., Kanda, Y., Yamaguchi, H., Osumi, M.: Electron microscope studies on the mechanism of action of clotrimazole on Candida albicans. Sabouraudia **11**, 205–209 (1973)

140 Iwata, K., Yamaguchi, H., Hiratani, T.: Mode of action of clotrimazole. Sabouraudia **11**, 158–166 (1973)

141 Jones, B. R., Clayton, Y. M., Jones, D. B., O'Day, D. M., Poirier, R. H.: The place of Canesten® in the management of oculomycosis. Münch. med. Wschr. **118**, Suppl. 1, 97–103 (1976)

141aKehrer, E., Brandt, G.: Mycoses in autopsy material: frequency, localization and causes. Mykosen **22**, 280–288 (1979)

142 Keller, K.: Klinische Erfahrungen mit dem neuen Antimykotikum Econazol. Schweiz. Rundsch. Med. (Praxis) **63**, 722–724 (1974)

143 Kern, R.: Die Wirkung von Econazol auf Hefezellen. Diplomarbeit, Technische Hochschule Darmstadt, 1976

144 Kern, R., Zimmermann, F. K.: Über dem Wirkungsmechanismus des Antimyzetikum Econazol. Mykosen **20**, 133–146 (1977)

145 Kern, R., Zimmermann, F. K.: Physiological effects of econazol nitrate on yeast cells. International Symposium Medical Mycology, Flims, 1977. Mykosen, Suppl. 1, 339–345 (1978)

146 Kessler, H.-J.: In vitro-Untersuchungen zur Frage der Beeinflussung der antimikrobiellen Wirkung von Isoconazol-Nitrat durch Diflucortolon-valerianat. Personal communication 1977

147 Kim, Jong Min; Eun Hee Chul; Lee, Chang Woo; Kim, Hong Sik: A study on therapeutic evaluation with econazole in patients with dermatomycoses and in vitro determination of minimal inhibitory concentration. Kor. J. Dermatol. **15**, 9–13 (1977)

148 Kligman, A.: The identification of contact allergens by human assay. J. invest. Derm. **47**, 369–374 (1966)

149 Kligman, A.: Personal communication. Contribution to the AAD Meeting, Chicago, 1976

150 Knapp, A., Hauff, U., Schwenke, W.: Über ein neues Antimykotikum auf Hydroxychinolinbasis. Derm. Wschr. **163**, 471–477 (1977)

151 Knüsel, H.: Vulvovaginale Mykosen – Kurztherapie (3 Tage) mit Econazol. Geburtsh. u. Frauenheilk. **37**, 43–47 (1977)

152 Konopka, E. A., Kimble, E. F., Zoganas, H. C., Heymann, H.: Antimicrobial effec-

tiveness of Locacorten-Vioform® cream in secondary infections of common dermatoses. Dermatologica (Basel) **151**, 1–8 (1975)

153 Korte, W., Senft, H. H.: Aktuelle topische Therapie der Genitalmykosen – vergleichende klinische Prüfung von Clotrimazol und Miconazol. Münch. med. Wschr. **118**, Suppl. 1, 45–48 (1976)

154 Krause, H.: Zur Behandlung der Trichonocardiosis palmellina mit Econazolnitrat-Spray. Arzneimittel-Forsch. **28**, 1804–1805 (1978)

155 Kuli, E.: Lokale Behandlung von Pilzaffektionen der Haut und der Nägel mit Daktarin®, einem neuen Breitspektrum-Antimykotikum. Schweiz. Rundsch. Med. (Praxis) **61**, 1308–1310 (1972)

156 Kunicke, A.: Ergebnisse der Clotrimazol-Therapie bei Candida- und Trichomonas-Infektionen. Arzneimittel-Forsch. **24**, 534–539 (1974)

157 Lambert, D., Chapuis, J. L., Camerlynck, P.: Devant la fréquence croissante des mycoses cutanées: Action de Pévaryl® en dermatologie, premiers résultats. Lyon méd. **237**, 353–354 (1977)

158 Lambotte, R., Dogniez, B., Sandront-Degee, M.: Influence of rectal infections caused by Candida albicans on the therapeutic results obtained in vaginal candidosis. International Symposium Medical Mycology, Flims, 1977. Mykosen, Suppl. 1, 311–313 (1978)

159 Lang, E.: Antibiotika-Therapie. München: Banaschewski 1975

160 Lang, E.: Anaerobe Infektionen. Antibiotika in der Praxis (Wien) **3**, 34–37 (1977)

161 Lange, H., Paetzold, O.-H., Grauer, E. K.: Antibiotikaresistenz von Staphylokokken bei Hauterkrankungen. Hautarzt **28**, 314–318 (1977)

162 Levine, H. B.: R 34000, a dioxolane imidazole in the therapy for experimental coccidioidomycosis. Chest **70**, 755–759 (1976)

163 Levine, H. B.: Econazole in experimental coccidioidomycosis. Curr. Chemother. **1978**, 233–234

164 Levine, H. B., Cobb, J. M.: Oral therapy for experimental coccidioidomycosis with R 41400 (ketoconazole), a new imidazole. Amer. Rev. resp. Dis. **118**, 715–721 (1978)

165 Levine, H. B., Stevens, D. A., Cobb, J. M., Gebhardt, A. E.: Miconazole in coccidioidomycosis. I. Assays of activity in mice and in vitro. J. infect. Dis. **132**, 407–413 (1975)

166 Leyden, J. J., Kligman, A. M.: The case for steroid-antibiotic combinations. Brit. J. Dermat. **96**, 179–187 (1977)

167 Lorente, F., Fontan, G., Garcia Rodriguez, M. C., Ojeda, J. A.: Treatment of chronic mucocutaneous candidiasis with imidazole derivatives. J. Pediat. **90**, 847 (1977)

168 Lorenzetti, O. J., Wernet, T. C.: Topical parabens: benefits and risks. Dermatologica (Basel) **154**, 244–250 (1977)

169 Lurie, D.: Die 3-Tage-Therapie der vaginalen Candidiasis. Ther. Umsch. **34**, 544–546 (1977)

170 Male, O.: Die Mykosetherapie im Alltag des Dermatologen. Z. Haut u. Geschl.-Kr. **52**, 237–238 (1976)

171 Male, O., Tappeiner, J.: Lokalanwendung von Econazol-Creme bei Dermatomykosen. Bericht über die klinische Prüfung bei 69 Fällen. Z. Haut- u. Geschl.-Kr. **52**, 1135–1141 (1977)

172 Marcionelli, L.: Terapia con ovuli all'econazolo da 150 mg della vulvovaginite fungina. Riv. Med. Svizz. Ital. **42**, 499–502 (1977)

173 Marmion, L. C., Desser, K. B., Lilly, R. B., Stevens, D. A.: Reversible thrombocytosis and anemia due to miconazole therapy. Antimicrobial Agents Chemother. **10**, 447–449 (1976)

174 Marples, M. J.: The normal flora of the human skin. Brit. J. Derm. **81**, Suppl. 1, 2–13 (1969)

175 Marples, R. R.: Local infections – experimental aspects. J. Soc. Cosmet. Chem. **27**, 449–457 (1976)

176 Marples, R. R., Rebora, A., Kligman, A. M.: Topical steroid-antibiotic combinations. Arch. Derm. **108**, 237–240 (1973)

177 Marsh, P. D., Selwyn, S.: Studies on antagonism between human skin bacteria. J. med. Microbiol. **10**, 161–169 (1977)

178 Martin-DuPan, R.: La mycose chez l'enfant. Le point de vue du pédiatre. Schweiz. Rundschau Med. (Praxis) **66**, 1461–1466 (1977)

179 Meberg, A., Langslet, A., Søvde, A., Kolstad, A.: Candida-septicemia with chorioretinitis, osteomyelitis and arthritis treated with systemic miconazole and intraarticular amphotericin B. Mykosen **20**, 257–260 (1977)

180 Mehnert, B., Schiefer, B.: Wechselseitige Beziehungen von Candida albicans und Staphylococcus aureus im Infektionsgeschehen. Vortrag 4. wissenschaftliche Tagung der deutschsprachigen mykologischen Gesellschaft, 119–123. Berlin-Heidelberg-New York: Springer 1967

181 Meinhof, W.: Angeborene Immundefektsyndrome und Candida-Mykose. Münch. med. Wschr. **118**, Suppl. 1, 3–5 (1976)

182 Meinhof, W.: Candida-Mykosen und celluläre Immundefekte. Zbl. Haut- und Geschl.-Kr. **141**, 1–10 (1979)

183 Meinhof, W., Schröpl, F.: Die Häufigkeit von hautpathogenen Pilzen bei Patienten einer überregionalen Diagnoseklinik. Ein Beitrag zur Epidemiologie der Dermatomykosen. Hautarzt **25**, 139–142 (1974)

184 Mermet, D., Long, B., Saad-Zoy, R.: Une affection d'actualité: Les mycoses vulvovaginales, leur traitement par un fongicide: l'éconazole. Premiers résultats. Lyon méd. **237**, 251–252 (1977)

185 Mertens, R. L. J., Morais, J., Verhamme, G.: A doubleblind study comparing Daktacort®, miconazole and hydrocortisone in inflammatory skin infections. Dermatologica (Basel) **153**, 228–235 (1976)

186 Meynadier, J., Guilhou, J. J., Meynadier, J.: Dermatoses d'actualité: les mycoses cutanées, un nouveau traitment: l'éconazole. Rev. Méditerr. Sci. Méd. **6**, 465–467 (1977)

187 Möller, C., Blumqvist, K., Kiviluoto, O.: Mykologische Flora des Anorektum. Mykosen **20**, 305–308 (1977)

188 Moreau, F., Dompmartin, D., Drouhet, E.: Essai de traitment, par un nouvel antifongique éconazole, sur des épidermomycoses tropicales. 6th Congress ISHAM, Tokyo, 1975

189 Moroff, H.: Erfahrungen bei der Behandlung der Genitalmykose mit einem neuen Antimykotikum in zwei verschiedenen Anwendungsformen. Inauguraldissertation, Göttingen 1975

190 Müller, J.: Pilzinfektionen im Gefolge antibiotischer Therapie. Münch. med. Wschr. **118**, 669–672 (1976)

191 Neldner, K. H.: The halogenated 8-hydroxyquinolines. Int. J. Dermat. **16**, 267–273 (1977)

192 Netter, A.: Progrès récents dans le traitment des candidoses vulvovaginales. Rév. franç. Gynéc. **72**, 237–240 (1977)

193 Neubert, U., Braun-Falco, O.: Mazeration der Zehenzwischenräume und gramnegativer Fußinfekt. Hautarzt **27**, 538–543 (1976)

194 Nielsen, M. L., Raahave, D., Stage, J. G., Justesen, T.: Anaerobic and aerobic skin bacteria before and after skin disinfection with chlorhexidine: An experimental study in volunteers. J. clin. Path. **28**, 793–797 (1975)

195 Nilsson, E., Henning, C.: The bacteriological flora in candidosis of the skin. Curr. ther. Res. **22**, 27–32 (1977)

196 Noble, W. C.: Variation in the prevalence of antibiotic resistance of Staphylococcus aureus from human skin and nares. J. gen. Microbiol. **98**, 125–132 (1977)

197 Nolte, H., Eggensperger, H.: Die Wirkung von Intimpflegemitteln aus mikrobiologischer Sicht. Ärztl. Kosmetol. **6**, 192–200 (1976)

198 Nolting, S., Fegeler, K.: Klinische Mykologie. Münch. med. Wschr. **120**, 1383–1384 (1978)
199 Nørgaard, O.: Pecilocinum-Allergie. Hautarzt **28**, 35–36 (1977)
200 Obolensky, W., Maire, F.: Die vulvo-vaginale Mykose und ihre Behandlung mit Econazol. Dtsch. med. Wschr. **100**, 1730–1733 (1975)
201 Obolensky, W., Maire, F.: Les mycoses vulvo-vaginales et leur traitement à l'éconazole. Méd. et Hyg. (Genève) **34**, 1913–1915 (1976)
202 Olschewski, M., Bickmann, M., Stolp, W., Patt, V., Schneider, J.: Untersuchungen zur Pharmakokinetik von Econazol bei vaginaler Applikation. Forschungsbericht, gynäkologische Klinik der Universität Bonn, BRD, 1973
203 Pap, J., Milakov, J.: Die Ergebnisse der klinischen Prüfung von Pevaryl Spray-Lösung 1% als Therapeutikum der lokalen Dermatomykosen. Schweiz. Rundschau Med. (Praxis) **67**, 652–654 (1978)
204 Park, Y. S., Yoo, H.: The clinical effects of three-day therapy for candidal vaginitis with econazole nitrate (150 mg) vaginal suppository. Kor. J. Obstet. Gynec. **21**, 201–204 (1978)
205 Parran, J., Brinkman, J., Brinkman, R. E.: The effect of human skin surface lipids upon the activity of antimicrobial agents. J. invest. Derm. **45**, 89–95 (1965)
206 Pastel, A., Taub, R., Zara, A.: Nouvel abord thérapeutique des mycoses cutanéomuqueuses. Sem. Hôp. (Paris) **52**, 549–552 (1976)
207 Patschke, K., Wegner, L. A., Oberste-Lehn, H., Horster, F. A.: Pharmakokinetische Untersuchungen nach topischer Anwendung von Clotrimazol (Canesten®). Münch. med. Wschr. **118**, Suppl. 1, 12–15 (1976)
208 Patt, V.: Hormonal contraception and vaginal mycoses. International Symposium Medical Mycology, Flims 1977, Mykosen, Suppl. 1, 258–266 (1978)
209 Peeters, F., Snauwaert, R., Van Cutsem, J., Amery, W.: A controlled trial with miconazole in the prevention of yeast infections occurring after treatment of vaginal trichomoniasis. Europ. J. Gyn. Reprod. Biol. **4**, 95–99 (1974)
210 Peios, E.: Lokalbehandlung von Soor-Kolpitis mit Econazol. Schweiz. Rundsch. Med. (Praxis) **64**, 1261–1262 (1975)
211 Perruchoud, A., Kobza, K., Kopp, C., Mihatsch, M., Herzog, H.: Klinik und Therapie der Candidiasis bei pneumologischen Patienten. Schweiz. med. Wschr. **107**, 192–194 (1977)
212 Pettit, J. H. S.: Treatment of superficial fungal infections of the skin. Drugs **10**, 130–142 (1975)
213 Pinault, L., Crestian, J.: Les médicaments vétérinaires antifongiques. 1. Substances de synthèse. Rec. Méd. vét. **154**, 419–424 (1978)
214 Plempel, M.: Probleme der Therapie mit modernen Antimykotika. Münch. med. Wschr. **118**, Suppl. 1, 19–23 (1976)
215 Plempel, M.: Wirkungen, Nebenwirkungen und Indikationen zweier neuer Azol-Antimykotika. Z. Hautkrankh. **52**, 242 (1977)
216 Plempel, M., Bartmann, K.: Experimentelle Untersuchungen zur antimykotischen Wirkung von Clotrimazol in vitro und bei lokaler Applikation in vivo. Arzneimittel-Forsch. **22**, 1280–1289 (1972)
217 Poitschek, C., Thurner, J., Haller, I.: Bestimmung der antimikrobiellen Wirksamkeit einer Kombination aus Azidamfenicol, Clotrimazol und Dexamethason in vitro. Arzneimittel-Forsch. **28**, 232–234 (1978)
218 Polenghi, F., Lasagni, A.: Observations on a case of mycokeratitis and its treatment with Bay b 5097 (Canesten®). Mykosen **19**, 223–226 (1976)
219 Poplack, D. G., Jacobs, S. A.: Candida arthritis treated with amphotericin B. J. Pediat. **87**, 989–990 (1975)
220 Preusser, H.-J.: Die Wirkung von Econazol auf die Feinstruktur der Zellen von Trichophyton rubrum, Mykosen **18**, 453–465 (1975)
221 Preusser, H.-J.: Effects of in vitro treatment with econazole on the ultrastructure of Candida albicans. Mykosen **19**, 304–316 (1976)

222 Preusser, H.-J.: Die Wirkung von Econazol-nitrat auf Candida albicans. II. Der Einfluß auf die Ultrastruktur der in-vivo-Zellen. Symposium über Econazol-nitrat, Boppard/Rhein 1977, pp. 41–47. Melsungen: Notabene Medici 1978

223 Preusser, H.-J., Rostek, H.: An unusual method of reproduction of Candida albicans and Trichophyton rubrum electron micrographs. Castellania 5, 87–90 (1977)

224 Preusser, H.-J., Rostek, H.: Pathogenesis of Candida albicans cells after treatment with econazole. Electron microscopic in vivo studies. Proceedings of the VIIth Congress of the International Society for Human and Animal Mycology, Tel Aviv, March 1979. Amsterdam: Excerpta Medica 1980 (in press).

225 Preusser, H.-J., Rostek, H., Einbeck, R.: Freeze-fracture studies of the plasma-lemma of Candida albicans after treatment with econazole nitrate. Sabouraudia 1980 (in press).

226 Privat, Y.: Face à la fréquence croissante des mycoses cutanées. Un nouveau fongi-cide polyvalent: l'éconazole. Sem. Hôp. Paris Thérapeutique 53, 153–155 (1977)

227 Privat, Y.: Traitement des dermatomycoses à composante inflammatoire par une association éconazole triamcinolone. Méditerranée médical 161, 77–78 (1978)

228 Qadripur, S. A., Bosse, K.: Econazol, ein neues Breitbandantimykotikum. Z. Haut. u. Geschle.-Kr. 49, 769–773 (1974)

229 Raab, W.: Die gegenseitige Beeinflussung von Tuberkulose und systemischer Moni-liasis. Derm. Wschr. 149, 401–408 (1964)

230 Raab, W.: Die immunologische Bedeutung mikrobieller Organismen an der Haut-oberfläche. Allergie u. Asthma 15, 222–228 (1969)

231 Raab, W.: Probleme der lokalen Corticosteroidbehandlung. Heidelberg: Hüthig 1971

232 Raab, W.: Dermatologie. Grundlagen und Praxis. Stuttgart: Fischer 1972

233 Raab, W.: Natamycin. Its properties and possibilities in medicine. Stuttgart: Thieme 1972. German Edition 1974

234 Raab, W.: Klinische Biochemie des Schocks. Stuttgart: Fischer 1975

235 Raab, W.: Effects of local corticosteroids in skin infections. Dermatologica (Basel) 152, Suppl. 1, 67–79 (1976)

236 Raab, W.: Untersuchungen zur Frage akuter unerwünschter Wirkungen von Erythromycin, Lincomycin und Clindamycin. Int. J. clin. Pharmacol. 15, 90–97 (1977)

237 Raab, W.: Clinical pharmacology of modern topical broad-spectrum antimicrobials. Curr. ther. Res. 22, 65–82 (1977)

238 Raab, W.: Spezifische und unspezifische Immunstimulation bei Herpes simplex recidivans. Z. Haut. u. Geschl.-Kr. 52, 565–572 (1977)

239 Raab, W.: Glucocorticoids and antimicrobials. International Symposium Medical Mycology, Flims, 1977. Mykosen, Suppl. 1, 304–310 (1978)

240 Raab, W.: Klinische Pharmakologie moderner Breitband-Antimykotika. Sympo-sion über Econazol-Nitrat, Boppard/Rhein, 1977, pp. 83–86. Melsungen: Nota-bene Medici 1978

241 Raab, W., Gmeiner, B.: Evaluation of econazole by Warburg assay; comparison with other antimicrobials. Mykosen 19, 238–240 (1976)

242 Raab, W., Gmeiner, B.: Interactions between econazole, a broad-spectrum antimi-crobic substance, and topically active glucocorticoids. Dermatologica (Basel) 153, 14–22 (1976)

243 Raab, W., Högl, F.: Enzyme inhibition by econazole and other antifungal imidazo-les. (In preparation).

244 Raab, W., Högl, F.: Interactions between imidazole antifungals and polyenes. (In preparation).

245 Raab, W., Högl, F.: The effect of econazole on rat liver mitochondria in vitro. (In preparation).

246 Raab, W., Killer, S.: Haloprogin. Seine Wirksamkeit in Gegenwart von Glukokorti-koiden und Neomycin. Z. Haut. u. Geschl.-Kr. 50, 499–505 (1975)

247 Raab, W., Kleinsorge, H.: Diagnose von Arzneimittelallergien. München-Berlin-Wien: Urban & Schwarzenberg 1968

248 Raab, W., Kleinsorge, H., Schwartz, N.: Arzneimittelallergien. Klinik, Diagnose, Differentialdiagnose und Therapie. Stuttgart: Fischer (in Vorbereitung)

249 Raab, W., Windisch, J.: In-vitro-Untersuchungen zur Anwendbarkeit von 1-p-Chlorbenzyl-2-methylbenzimidazol in der Mykosebehandlung. Arch. Derm. Forsch. **240**, 365–374 (1971)

250 Raab, W., Windisch, J.: Zur Entstehung der Candidosen nach Trichomonadenbehandlung. Z. Haut. u. Geschl.-Kr. **48**, 381–384 (1973)

251 Raab, W., Windisch, J. M.: Experimental study on interactions between fluocinonide, neomycin, gramicidin and nystatin. Castellania **3**, 51–58 (1975)

252 Randiandiche, M.: Fréquence de Pityrosporum ovale dans l'oreille humaine. Dermatologica (Basel) **151**, 100–103 (1975)

253 Refal, M.: Vergleichende Bewertung der antimyzetischen Wirkung von Miconazol in vitro und der antimykotischen Wirkung von Epi-Monistat® und Gyno-Monistat® in vivo. Rodenwaldt-Arch. **1**, 26–31 (1974)

254 Reyes-Javier, P.: Topical treatment of inflammatory dermatoses and cutaneous candidiasis with a new corticosteroid-antibiotic combination: halcinonide-neomycin-amphotericin. Brit. J. clin. Pract. **31**, 33–39 (1977)

255 Rieth, H.: Epidemiologie der Mykosen in Deutschland und Wandel im Erregerspektrum. Münch. med. Wschr. **118**, Suppl. 1, 69–75 (1976)

256 Rieth, H.: Die Rolle der Schimmelpilze in der Dermatologie. Z. Haut. u. Geschl.-Kr. **52**, 235–236 (1977)

257 Rindt, W., Geibel, W., Appel, L.: Untersuchungen zur vaginalen Resorption von Econazol. Arzneimittel-Forsch. **29**, 697–699 (1979)

258 Rohde, B.: Balanitis, eine Indikation für Ampho-Moronal-Lösung. Castellania **5**, 221–222 (1977)

259 Roller, J. A.: Contact allergy to clotrimazole. Brit. med. J. **1978/III**, 78

260 Roschke, W.: Die proktologische Sprechstunde. München: Urban & Schwarzenberg 1969

261 Roubicek, M., Krebs, A.: Logamel®, ein neues Lokaltherapeutikum bei infizierten entzündlichen Dermatosen. Ergebnisse einer kontrollierten Prüfung bei akuten Dermatomykosen. Schweiz. Rundsch. Med. (Praxis) **66**, 585–588 (1977)

262 Ruppen, N.: Therapie der Soorkolpitis mit Econazol. Schweiz. Rundsch. Med. (Praxis) **66**, 86–88 (1977)

263 Samsoen, M., Jelen, G.: Allergy to Daktarin gel. Contact Dermatitis **3**, 351–352 (1977)

264 Savage, C. A.: 2-, 4, 4'-Trichloro-2'-hydroxydiphenylether, a new bacteriostat, and its use in cosmetic products. 6. Congr. Int. Fed. Soc. Cosm. Chemists. Barcelona 1970. Drug Cosm. Indus. **109**, 36 (1971)

265 Sawyer, P. R., Brogden, R. N., Pinder, R. M., Speight, T. M., Avery, G. S.: Miconazole: a review of its antifungal activity and therapeutic efficacy. Drugs **9**, 406–423 (1975)

266 Sawyer, P. R., Brogden, R. N., Pinder, R. M., Speight, T. M., Avery, G. S.: Clotrimazole: a review of its antifungal activity and therapeutic efficacy. Drugs **9**, 424–447 (1975)

267 Schacter, I. P., Owellen, R. J., Rathbun, H. K., Buchanan, B.: Antagonism between miconazole and amphotericin B. Lancet **1976/II**, 318

268 Schaefer, H.: Pharmakokinetische Untersuchungen nach topischer Anwendung von Econazol-nitrat. Symposion über Econazol-nitrat. Boppard/Rhein 1977, pp. 87–100. Melsungen: Notabene Medici 1978

269 Schaefer, H., Stüttgen, G.: Biopharmaceutical problems in the treatment of superficial mycoses. International Symposium Medical Mycology, Flims, 1977. Mykosen, Suppl. 1, 164–170 (1978)

270 Schaefer, H., Stüttgen, G.: Absolute concentrations of an antimycotic agent, econ-

azole, in the human skin after local application. Arzneimittel-Forsch. **26**, 432–435 (1976)

271 Schär, G., Kayser, F. H., Dupont, M. C.: Antimicrobial activity of econazole and miconazole in vitro and in experimental candidiasis and aspergillosis. Chemotherapy **22**, 211–220 (1976)

272 Scherrer, M., Knüsel, F., Weirich, E. G.: Zur Kenntnis der antimikrobiellen Aktivität von Breitspektrum-Antimikrobika unter besonderer Berücksichtigung der Salicylsäure. Mykosen **14**, 323–334 (1971)

273 Scherwitz, C.: Candidaerkrankungen von Haut und Schleimhaut. Med. Klin. 71, 1172–1182 (1976)

274 Scherwitz, C.: Klinische Prüfung von Econazol Haut-Milch und -Creme bei Hautmykosen. Z. Haut. u. Geschl.-Kr. **52**, 117–125 (1977)

275 Schmid, P.: Klinische Erfahrungen bei der Behandlung von Hautmykosen mit Econazol-Crème und -Puder. Schweiz. Rundsch. Med. (Praxis) **63**, 1156–1158 (1974)

276 Schmid, P.: Zweiphasenbehandlung entzündlicher Hautmykosen mit Pevisone/Pevaryl. Schweiz. Rundsch. Med. (Praxis) **68**, 233–235 (1979)

277 Schnell, J. D.: Erfahrungen mit dem Antimykotikum Bay b 5097 bei der lokalen Behandlung der Trichomonas vaginalis Infektion. Geburtsh. u. Frauenheilk. **32**, 787–790 (1972)

278 Schnell, J. D., Plempel, M.: Verhütung des Neugeborenen-Soor durch antepartale Behandlung der Mutter. Münch. med. Wschr. **118**, Suppl. 1, 35–37 (1976)

279 Schnell, J. D., Plempel, M., Kreysing, M.: Epidemiologie der Vaginalmykose in der Gravidität und ihre Bedeutung für das Neugeborene. Münch. med. Wschr. **118**, Suppl. 1, 30–32 (1976)

280 Scholer, H. J.: Grundlagen und Ergebnisse der antimykotischen Chemotherapie mit 5-Fluorocytosin. Chemotherapy **22**, Suppl. 1, 103–146 (1976)

281 Schuerwegh, W.: Clinical evaluation of econazole nitrate in 1% vaginal cream for treatment of vaginal candidosis. Europ. J. Obstet. Gynec. reprod. Biol. **8**, 5–7 (1978)

282 Schwarz, K. J., Much, Th., Konzelmann, M.: Poliklinische Prüfung von Econazol bei 594 Fällen von Hautmykosen. Dtsch. med. Wschr. **100**, 1497–1500 (1975)

283 Schwarz, K. J., Luggen, H., Bänninger, R., Konzelmann, M.: Poliklinische Prüfung von Pevisone. Doppelblindstudie an 101 Patienten. Schweiz. Rundschau Med. (Praxis) **67**, 1112–1116 (1978)

284 Schweisfurth, R.: Untersuchungen über den Effekt einer Econazol-Nitrat-Behandlung auf vaginale Laktobakterien. (In preparation)

285 Seki, S., Nomiya, B., Koeda, T., Umemura, K., Oda, M., Ogawa, H.: Laboratory evaluation of M-1028 (2,4,5-Trichlorophenyl-γ-iodopropargyl ether), a new antimicrobial agent. Antimicrobial Agents Chemother. **1963**, 569–572

286 Selwyn, S.: Natural antibiosis among skin bacteria as a primary defence against infection. Brit. J. Derm. **93**, 487–493 (1975)

287 Selwyn, S.: Bacterial vaginitis and the rationale of clotrimazole therapy. Münch. med. Wschr. **118**, Suppl. 1, 49–52 (1976)

288 Shreedhara Swamy, K. H., Sirst, M., Ramananda Rao, G.: Studies on the mechanism of action of miconazole: effect of miconazole on respiration and cell permeability of Candida albicans. Antimicrobial Agents Chemother. **5**, 420–425 (1973)

289 Siboulet, A.: L'éconazole spray-poudre en dermatovénérologie. Schweiz. Rundsch. Med. (Praxis) **65**, 977–981 (1976)

290 Spickhoff, H., Kreysing, W., Schnell, J. D.: Canesten®/Miconazol-Ovula, ein Vaginaltherapie-Vergleich. Münch. med. Wschr. **118**, Suppl. 1, 67–68 (1976)

291 Spiechowicz, E., Bak, Z., Bielunska, S.: Clinical evaluation of natamycin 2,5% suspension in the treatment of a denture stomatitis infected with Candida albicans. Castellania **5**, 175–180 (1977)

292 Spiekermann, P. H., Young, M. D., Bloomfield, N. J.: Clinical evaluation of clotrimazole. A broad-spectrum antifungal agent. Arch. Derm. **112**, 350–352 (1976)

293 Stahl, D., Onsberg, P.: Local treatment of dermatomycosis Mykosen **21**, 49–52 (1978)
294 Staib, F., Geier, R.: Proteolysis products of Candida albicans as a substrate for growth of Staphylococcus aureus – A preliminary report. Zbl. Bakt., I. Abt. Orig. A **218**, 374–375 (1971)
295 Staib, F., Grosse, G., Mishra, S. K.: Staphylococcus aureus and Candida albicans infection (animal experiments). Zbl. Bakt. I. Abt. Orig. A **234**, 450–461 (1976)
296 Stevens, D. A., Levine, H. B., Deresinski, S. C.: Miconazole in coccidioidomycosis. II. Therapeutic and pharmacologic studies in man. Amer. J. Med. **60**, 191–202 (1976)
297 Storck, H.: Experimentelle Untersuchungen zur Frage der Bedeutung von Mikroben in der Ekzemgenese. Dermatologica (Basel) **96**, 177–262 (1948)
298 Stuchlik, S.: Über die Behandlung von Soor-Mykosen bei Leukaemie-Patienten mit parenteral applizierbarem Miconazol. Med. Welt **26**, 1255–1256 (1975)
299 Stüttgen, G.: Quoted from Schwarz, K. J. et al. [282]
300 Stüttgen, G., Schaefer, H.: Funktionelle Dermatologie. Berlin-Heidelberg-New York: Springer 1976
301 Sturm, W., Gerlach, Ch.: Verträglichkeitsprüfung von Chlorhydroxychinolinen und klinische Erfahrungen mit einer Versuchsrezeptur. Derm. Wschr. **163**, 543–549 (1977)
302 Sung, J. P.: Treatment of disseminated coccidioidomycosis with miconazole. West. Med. **124**, 191–198 (1976)
303 Svejgaard, E.: Miconazole in the treatment of candidiasis of the digestive tract. Acta derm.-venereol. (Stockh.) **56**, 303–306 (1976)
304 Symoens, J.: Miconazole for the treatment of systemic mycosis: A review. IXth Int. Congress of Chemotherapy, London 1975
305 Szarmach, H., Poniecka, H., Stepka, L.: Clortrimazol in der Behandlung von Hautmykosen. Hautarzt **28**, 140–144 (1977)
305a Suter, L., Rabbat, M., Nolting, S.: Gramnegativer Fußinfekt. Mykosen **22**, 109–114 (1979)
306 Tausch, I.: Zur Wirksamkeit einiger Antimykotika. Derm. Wschr. **163**, 223–234 (1977)
306a Täuber, U.: Percutaneous absorption of isoconazole in humans. Mykosen **22**, 223–232 (1979)
306b Täuber, U., Rzadkiewicz, M.: Bioavailability of isoconazole in the skin. Mykosen **22**, 201–216 (1979)
307 Tennstedt, D., Lestienne, M. C., Wustfeld, A., Lachapelle, J. M.: Traitment du pied d'athlète en milieu industriel par le nitrate d'éconazole spray-poudre. Louvain méd. **96**, 441–445 (1977)
308 Tettenborn, D., Lorke, D., Machener, L.: Experimentelle toxikologische Untersuchungen mit Clotrimazol unter besonderer Berücksichtigung der Reproduktionstoxität und Neugeborenenverträglichkeit. Münch. med. Wschr. **118**, Suppl. 1, 24–26 (1976)
309 Thienpont, D., Van Cutsem, J., Van Nueten, J. M., Niemegeers, C. J. E., Marsboom, R.: Biological and toxicological properties of econazole, a broad-spectrum antimycotic. Arzneimittel-Forsch. **25**, 224–230 (1975)
310 Thienpont, D., Van Cutsem, J., Gough, D. A.: Treatment of gastrointestinal candidosis in predisposed guinea pigs and in conventional mice with miconazole. Mykosen **21**, 417–424 (1978)
310a Török, I., Várkonyi, V., Podányi, B., Soós, G.: Erfahrungen mit Mycosolon in der klinischen Anwendung. Derm. Mschr. **162**, 188–189 (1976)
310b Török, I., Várkonyi, V., Podányi, B., Soós, G., Dénes, M., Király, K.: Vergleichende Untersuchungen mit Mycosolon, Miconazol und Depersolon Salbe im Doppelblindversuch. Derm. Mschr. **165**, 788–794, (1979)
311 Toulouse, R., Taillanter, L.: Une affection gynécologique d'actualité: les candidoses

vulvo-vaginales. Un progrès décisif dans leur traitement: l'éconazole. L'Ouest Médical **30**, 1179–1182 (1977)

312 Utz, J. P.: New drugs for the systemic mycoses: flucytosine and clotrimazole. Bull. N. Y. Acad. Med. **51**, 1103–1108 (1975)

313 Van Cutsem, J. M., Thienpont, D. C.: Miconazole, a broad-spectrum antimycotic agent with antibacterial activity. Chemotherapy **17**, 392–404 (1972)

314 Vandaele, R., Uyttendaele, K.: Miconazole nitrate in the topical treatment of dermatomycoses. A clinical evaluation. Arzneimittel-Forsch. **22**, 1221–1223 (1972)

315 Van den Bossche, H.: Biochemical effects of miconazole on fungi. I. Effects on the uptake and/or utilization of purines, pyrimidines, nucleosides, amino acids and glucose by Candida albicans. Biochem. Pharmacol. **23**, 887–899 (1974)

316 Van den Bossche, H., Willemsens, G., Van Cutsem, J. M.: The action of miconazole on the growth of Candida albicans. Sabouraudia **13**, 63–73 (1975)

317 Van den Bossche, H., Willemsens, G., Cools, W., Lauwers, W. F. J., Lejeune, L.: Biochemical effects of miconazole on fungi. II. Inhibition of ergosterol synthesis in Candida albicans. Chem. Biol. Interact. **21**, 59–78 (1978)

318 Vanderdonckt, J., Lauwers, W., Bockaert, J.: Miconazole alcoholic solution in the treatment of mycotic nail infections. Mykosen **19**, 251–256 (1976)

319 Vandersarl, J. V., Sheppard, R. H.: Clotrimazole vs. haloprogin treatment of tinea cruris. Arch. Dermatol. **113**, 1233–1235 (1977)

320 Verma, B. S.: Econazole cream in fungal infections of the skin. Curr. ther. Res. **24**, 745–752 (1978)

321 Vogelsberg, H.: Klinische Erfahrungen bei Behandlung von Hautmykosen mit 1% Econazol Spray-Lösung und 1% Econazol Spray-Puder. Z. Hautkr. **53**, 648–650 (1978)

322 Voigt, W.-H.: Die Wirkung von Clotrimazol (Canesten®) auf die Ultrastruktur von Schimmelpilzen (Aspergillus fumigatus) im infizierten Tier. Mykosen **19**, 345–353 (1976)

323 Voigt, W.-H., Plempel, M.: Elektronenmikroskopische Untersuchungen an humanpathogenen Pilzen. I. Mitt.: Ultrastrukturelle Veränderungen von Candida albicans-Zellen durch Clotrimazol im Tierexperiment. Arzneimittel-Forsch. **24**, 508–515 (1974)

324 Voigt, W.-H., Schnell, J. D.: Elektronenmikroskopische Untersuchungen an humanpathogenen Pilzen. II. Mitt.: Ultrastrukturelle Veränderungen von Candida albicans-Zellen am menschlichen Vaginalepithel unter der Behandlung mit Clotrimazol. Arzneimittel-Forsch. **24**, 516–521 (1974)

325 Vukovich, A., Heald, A., Darragh, A.: Vaginal absorption of two imidazole antifungal agents, econazole and miconazole. Clin. Pharmacol. Ther. **21**, 121 (1977)

326 Wachs, G. N., Maibach, H. I.: Co-operative doubleblind trial of an antibiotic-corticoid combination in impetiginized atopic dermatitis. Brit. J. Derm. **95**, 323–328 (1976)

327 Wade, T. R., Jones, H. E., Chanda, J.: Efficacy of parenteral miconazole therapy in mycotic infection. Clin. Res. **25**, 287A (1977)

328 Walch, J.: Zur Behandlung der Hautmykosen. Schweiz. Rundschau Med. (Praxis) **67**, 1139–1143 (1978)

329 Wallace, S. M., Shah, V. P., Epstein, W. L., Greenberg, J.: Topically applied antifungal agents. Arch. Dermatol. **113**, 1539–1542 (1977)

330 Wallenburg, H. C. S., Wladimiroff, J. W.: Recurrence of vulvovaginal candidosis during pregnancy. Comparison of miconazole vs. nystatin treatment. Obstet. and Gynec. **48**, 491–494 (1976)

331 Ward-Jenkins, J.: Quoted from Roller, J. A. [259]

332 Warren, R. M., Welply, G. A. C., Elstein, M.: The treatment of vaginal candidosis. A comparative trial of miconazole, amphotericin and povidone iodine. Clin. Trials J. **11**, 148–151 (1974)

333 Welbourne, E., Champion, R. H., Parish, W. E.: Hypersensitivity to bacteria in eczema. I. Brit. J. Derm. **94**, 619–632 (1976)

332a Weitgasser, H., Herms, E.: Comparative clinical investigations with the new antimycotic agent isoconazole nitrate and its combination with diflucortolone-21-valerate in the case of inflammatory and eczematised dermatomycoses. Mykosen **22**, 177–183 (1979)

334 Wente, W.: Pyrrolnitrin zur Behandlung von Dermatomakosen und dem Erythrasma in der dermatologischen Praxis. Mykosen **20**, 463–470 (1977)

335 Wenzel-Heiniger, K.: Beitrag zur Therapie der vulvo-vaginalen Mykosen. Schweiz. Rundsch. Med. (Praxis) **65**, 287–288 (1976)

336 Wersten, D.: Zur therapeutischen Anwendung antimykotischer Substanzen. Schweiz. med. Wschr. **106**, 455–459 (1976)

337 Wrigley, P. F. M., Tobias, J. S., Shaw, E.: Combination antifungal therapy for cryptococcal meningitis. Postgrad. med. J. **52**, 305–308 (1976)

338 Yamaguchi, H., Iwata, K.: Mechanism of action of clotrimazole and miconazole on the mycotic cell wall. 18th General Meeting of the Japanese Society of Medical Mycology, Tokyo 1974

339 Yamaguchi, H., Iwata, K.: Studies on the membrane-active properties of imidazole antymycoties: Selective sensibility of lecithin liposomes depending on their lipid composition. VIIth Congress of the International Society for Human and Animal Mycology, Tel Aviv, March 1979

340 Yamasaki, Y., Uchida, K., Yamaguchi, H., Hiratani, T., Yamamoto, Y., Iwata, K.: Studies on antifungal activities of econazole 1. In vitro antimicrobial activity. Japan. J. med. Mycol. **18**, 216–224 (1977)

341 Zaias, N., Battistini, F.: Superficial mycoses. Treatment with a new broad-spectrum antifungal agent: 1% clotrimazole solution. Arch. Derm. **113**, 307–308 (1977)

342 Zazgornik, J., Schmidt, P., Thurner, J., Kopsa, H., Deutsch, E.: Klinik und Therapie der Pilzinfektionen nach Nierentransplantation. Dtsch. med. Wschr. **100**, 2082–2093 (1975)

343 Zimmermann, F. K.: The permeabilizing effect of econazole nitrate on yeast cells. 6th Congress ISHAM, Tokyo, 1975

344 Zimmermann, F. K., Kern, R.: Genetic aspects of medical mycology. International Symposium Medical Mycology, Flims, 1977. Mykosen, Suppl. 1, 36–42 (1978)

345 Baran, R., Beury, J., Civatte, J., Desmons, F., Hincky, M., Meynadier, J., Moulin, G., Privat, Y., Thivolet, J.: Etude thérapeutique multicentrique d'une nouvelle association d'un antifongique à large spectre et d'un corticoide. Sem. Hop. Paris **55**, 269–272 (1979)

346 Clayton, Y. M., Gange, R. W., Macdonals, D. M., Carruthers, J. A.: clinical double-blind trial of topical haloprogin and miconazole against superficial fungal infections. Clin. Exp. Dermat. **4**, 65–73 (1979)

347 Hesseling, W., Weuta, H.: Ekzemtherapie mit Baycuten und Baycuten SD. Wirkung und Verträglichkeit. Med. Welt **30**, 581–586 (1979)

348 Hoeprich, P. D.: New antifungal drugs in the therapy of systemic mycoses. Scand. J. Infect. Dis. Suppl. **16**, 74–79 (1978)

349 Kennedy, C.: Gram-negative folliculitis of the face. Clin. Exp. Dermat. **4**, 123–124 (1979)

350 Lecart, C., Clearhout, F., Franck, R., Godts, P., Lilien, C., Macours, L., Schuerwegh, W., Longrée, H., Mine, M., Strebelle, P., Van Gijsegem, M., Wesel, S.: A new treatment of vaginal candidiasis: three-day treatment with econanzole. Europ. J. Obstet. Gynec. Reprod. Biol. **9**, 125–127 (1979)

351 Loiudice, L., Lucisano, F.: Terapia a breve termine della candidiasi vaginale con un nuovo derivato imidazolico. Atti della Accademia Medica Lombarda **32**, 1–7 (1977)

352 Leyden, J. J., Stewart, R., Kligman, A. M.: Updated in vivo methods for evaluating

topical antimicrobial agents on human skin. J. Invest. Dermatol. **72**, 165–170 (1979)

353 Thong, Y. H., Ferrante, A.: Miconazole prolongs murine skin graft survival. Clin. Exp. Immunol. **35**, 10–12 (1979)

354 Preusser, H.-J., Rostek, H., Klein, M., Becker, H., Nass, W. P.: Elektronenmikroskopische Untersuchungen an Candida albicans aus vaginalem Abstrichmaterial während einer 3-Tage-Therapie mit Econazol. Arzneimittel-Forsch. **29**, 1432–1437 (1979)

355 Wendt, H., Kessler, J.: Antimikrobielle Wirksamkeit des Breitspektrum-Antimykotikums Isoconazolnitrat im Humanversuch. Arzneimittel-Forsch. **29**, 846–848 (1979)

356 Jevons, S., Gymer, G. E., Brammer, K. W., Cox, D. A., Leeming, M. R. G.: Antifungal activity of tioconazole (UK-20, 349), a new imidazole derivative. Antimicrobial Agents Chemother. **15**, 597–602 (1979)

357 Svendsen, E., Lie, S., Gunderson, Th., Lyngstad-Vik, I., Skuland, J.: Comparative evaluation of miconazole, clotrimazole and nystatin in the treatment of candidal vulvovaginitis. Curr. Ther. Res. **23**, 666–672 (1978)

358 Sauer, H.: Kombinationsbehandlung genitoanaler Ekzeme mit Baycuten und Baycuten SD. Therapiewoche **29**, (27) 53–54 (1979)

17 Subject Index

154

G. Plewig, A. M. Kligman

Acne

Morphogenesis and Treatment

1975. 110 plates, mostly in color. XII, 333 pages
ISBN 3-540-07212-8

Acne vulgaris is an extraordinarily common disease, found throughout the world. Some see the disorder as merely cosmetic. Nonetheless, few skin diseases cause as much physical and psychological misery as this scourge of adolescence. Dermatologists of course have more than a passing familiarity with acne vulgaris. Recognition is easy, but there is still an extraordinary amout of controversy concerning causative factors and the best modes of treatment. Recent advances have brought forth some important illuminations about which practicing physicians know too little.
This book offers the first complete account of the great diversity of clinical expressions. Moreover, gross morphology is coordinated with a thorough microscopic analysis of evolution of the disease. The material is presented in a readable and stimulating way. References are limited because they have been carefully selected.
This work with its many color illustrations, being intended for physicians who care for acne patients, is above all a practical treatise to assist doctors to diagnose and treat acne, and not only acne vulgaris but all the species of acne. The entire acne problem is reviewed, with contributions from bacteriology, endocrinology, physiology, anatomy, immunology, cellular kinetics and experimantal acne. The book concludes with an optimistic presentation of therapeutic strategic which make it possible for the informed physician to control the effects of this distressing disorder.

Contents: A Precise of Pathogenesis. – The Anatomy of Follicles. – Sebaceous Glands. – Bacteriology. – The Evolution of the Comedo. – The Dynamics of Primary Comedo Formation. – The Dynamics of Secondary Comedo Formation. – The Dynamics of Inflammation. – Inflammatory Lesions and Sequellae. – Classification of Acne Vulgaris. – Acne Conglobata. – Masculinizing Syndromes. – Gram-Negative Folliculitis. – Acne Neonatorum. – Acne Excoriée des Jeunes Filles. – Premenstrual Acne. – Post Adolescent Acne of the Back. – Acne Mechanica. – Acne Cosmetica. – Pomade Acne. – Acne Detergicans. – Acne and Acneiform Eruptions. – Acne Venenata. – Steroid Acne. – Acne Aestivalis (Mallorca Acne). – Rosacea. – The Role of Demodex. – Treatment – General Statement. – Spontaneous Involution of Acne. – Author Index. – Subject Index.

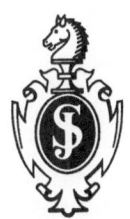

Springer-Verlag
Berlin
Heidelberg
New York

Springer
Dermatology

A Selection

O. Braun-Falco, H. Goldschmidt,
S. Lukacs

Dermatalogic Radiotherapy

1976. 48 figures, including 16 color
plates. XIV, 154 pages
ISBN 3-540-90186-8

V. M. Der Kaloustian, A. K. Kurban

Genetic Diseases of the Skin

With a Foreword by F. Clarke Fraser

1979. 441 figures, 17 tables.
XIII, 339 pages
ISBN 3-540-09151-3

S. Fregert, H.-J. Bandmann

Patch Testing

On behalf of the International Contact
Dermatitis Research Group. With contributions by numerous experts

1975. 3 figures, 17 tables. V, 78 pages
ISBN 3-540-07229-2

J. Petres, M. Hundeiker

Dermatosurgery

With a foreword by K. W. Kalkoff. Trans
lation from the German

1978. 112 figures. XVII, 152 pages
ISBN 3-540-90296-1

Physical Modalities in Dermatologic Therapy

Radiotherapy – Electrosurgery – Photo-
therapy – Cryosurgery.

Editor: H. Goldschmidt

1978. 317 figures, (16 in color), 62 tables
XV, 290 pages
ISBN 3-540-90267-8

B. Schaumann, M. Alter

Dermatoglyphics in Medical Disorders

1976. 74 figures, 51 tables. XI, 258 page:
ISBN 3-540-07555-0

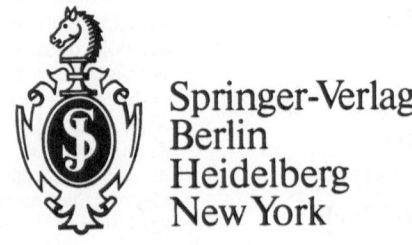

Springer-Verlag
Berlin
Heidelberg
New York